THE KOOK'S GUIDE TO SURFING
THE ULTIMATE INSTRUCTION MANUAL: HOW TO RIDE WAVES WITH SKILL, STYLE, AND ETIQUETTE

Jason Borte

Skyhorse Publishing

ABOUT THE AUTHOR

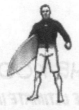

Jason Borte's first book, *Pipe Dreams: A Surfer's Journey* (HarperEntertainment 2003), appeared on the *New York Times* bestseller list for hardcover nonfiction. A former editor for *Surfer, Surfing, Explorations*, and Swell.com, he has also written features for *Eastern Surf, Transworld Surf Business, Water, Mundo Rad, Flow* (Japan), *Tripsurf* (France), *Adrenalin* (England), and *Australian Surfing Life*. Most recently, his work appeared in *The Mountain and the Wave, The Quiksilver Story* (Chronicle 2006), *The Best of Surfer Magazine* (Chronicle 2007), and *Pipeline: The World's Most Respected Wave* (Surfline 2008).

ACKNOWLEDGMENTS

To Mom and Dad for being supportive of my habit.

To Steve Hawk for the opportunity and guidance.

To the guys who showed me how to not be a kook—
Wes, Pillsbury, Kochey, Quest, Cuppa Joe, MJ, Twig, Ken,
Avery, Kliney, Cab, Neff, Greek, Brad, Brad, Jesse, Smitty,
Jimbo, Jeff, and Zeke.

To Scott the Lifeguard, Amy Beach, Don Spencer, and
Keegan for their work on this book.

To KV, Geebs, Lil' Ballurfin' Momma, and the Hudster for
keeping me honest.

And to Derrick for leading me to surfing and making me
write this book.

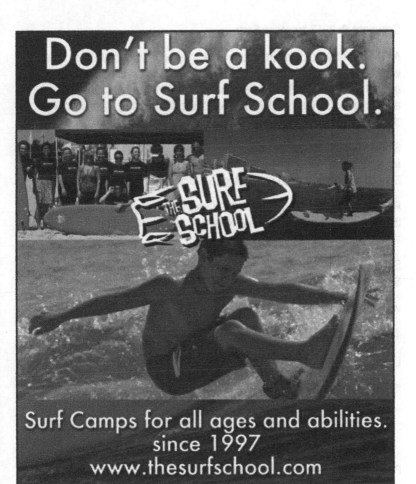

Skyhorse Publishing books may be purchased in bulk at special discounts for sales promotion, corporate gifts, fund-raising, or educational purposes. Special editions can also be created to specifications.

For details, contact the Special Sales Department, Skyhorse Publishing, 307 West 36th Street, 11th Floor, New York, NY 10018 or info@skyhorsepublishing.com.

Skyhorse® and Skyhorse Publishing® are registered trademarks of Skyhorse Publishing, Inc.®, a Delaware corporation.

www.skyhorsepublishing.com

10 9 8 7 6 5 4 3 2

Library of Congress Cataloging-in-Publication Data is available on file.

ISBN: 978-1-62087-723-4

Printed in the United States of America

TABLE OF CONTENTS

PART IV: MANEUVERS

PART VI: APPENDICES

INTRODUCTION

Surfing has been around for thousands of years, and more people surf today than at any time in history. Recent estimates put the number of current wave riders in the neighborhood of twenty million. Participants come from every walk of life, age, color, religion, and socioeconomic status. Twenty million seems like a significant number until you consider that is only around ⅓ percent of all earthlings. To the rest of the world's population, the other 99.7 percent, surfing remains misunderstood and misrepresented, and riding waves is considered a waste of time.

Who is to blame for surfing's bad rap? I say it's the kooks. In layman's terms, a kook is a person who is slightly off-the-wall, or something of a screwball. In surfing jargon, a kook really doesn't get it. Beginning surfers are considered kooks, but fortunately anyone can learn to surf. Having taught three-year-olds just out of diapers and seventy-year-olds soon to return to diapers, I truly believe that any able-bodied individual can learn to ride waves on his or her own. Developing proficiency in surfing marks step one on the road out of Kookville, but we cannot ride these mere skills off into the sunset. Plenty of avid, competent surfers remain full-fledged kooks. More than a novice at riding waves, a kook behaves in a manner that insults surfers and non-surfers alike. These people are oblivious to their transgressions and perpetuate surfing's negative stereotype. Kooks are the bad apples that spoil the bunch.

One trait of a kook is overuse of the word "dude." Society pigeonholes the speaker of this word as a surfer faster than screaming "jihad" marks one as a militant Muslim. A good friend of mine, a total landlubber, finds a way to fit "dude" into nearly every sentence he speaks. He does not surf, yet people wrongly label him as such. He gets branded as "that surfer dude" without ever dipping so much as his little toe in the surf.

The surfing stereotype was set in stone with Jeff Spicoli, the quintessential stoned surfer played by Sean Penn in the 1982 teen epic *Fast Times at Ridgemont High.* Of the thousands of surfers who I know, most only use the word "dude" to make a mockery of those who do. Nevertheless, if you surf, society assumes you have no real job, you make no money, and you spend your days hanging around the beach. I hate the beach, and the sun for that matter. I tolerate both as necessary evils in order to surf.

Thanks to the perpetuation of surfer as punk, loser, and burnout, surfing has been unable to rise above its lowly status. I, for one, do not believe that surfers are bums. Therefore, I set out a few years ago to change the "surfer dude" image. I contacted both the "Dummies" and "Idiots" guides about publishing a manual for the masses, a book that would explain not just surfing but how to be a surfer. Both the Dummies and Idiots declined, clinging to the old-school mentality that surfing was too unconventional to warrant the investment. Surfers, they assumed, do not read books. Whether surfers read books or not missed the point. Remember, 99.7 percent of the population does not surf.

Surfers cannot be herded into any category. They share an affinity for riding waves, but beyond that they go their separate ways. Unfortunately, since there are relatively few of us, we all automatically represent surfing. Our actions, good or bad, define surfing to outsiders.

In all the books I have seen on surfing (and there seems to be a new one published each week), I have not come across one that adequately explains how to be a responsible surfer as opposed to how to be a stereotypical surfer. These manuals overemphasize the spiritual and metaphysical aspects of communing with nature and fail to explain the process in simple terms, like you would with any other pursuit.

My goal is to teach you how to surf, but also to show you how to be a responsible surfer. How, in other words, not to be a kook.

I hope to achieve two goals with this book. First, I want you to abandon the "legions of the unjazzed," as '60s California icon Phil Edwards dubbed those people who have not experienced the joys of surfing. Riding waves is not that difficult. Quit making excuses and get out there. Second, when you surf, be cool. Not cool as in, "I'm a surfer and I'm too cool for school," but in terms of being accountable for your actions and considerate of others. The surf is a crowded place, and there is no room out there for kooks. I want you to become a responsible, respectable practitioner of the most enjoyable pursuit on the planet. Who knows, maybe I will see you in the water one day. If so, please don't be a kook. I promise to do the same. ✳

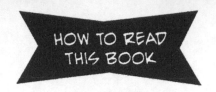

HOW TO READ THIS BOOK

THIS BOOK IS DIVIDED INTO SEVEN PARTS.

Part I, Basic Surfology, provides an explanation of what surfing is as well as a step-by-step guide describing how to do it. It also includes important chapters on fitness, dangers, and etiquette. If you have never surfed, I strongly urge you to read all of Part I before getting in the water.

From there, *Parts II and III* explore waves and equipment. While not required reading for your first session, they provide valuable insight. Maneuvers are broken down in *Part IV,* followed by *Organized Surfing in Part V.* Each of these can wait until you have surfed for a while and are starting to get the hang of it. *Finally, Part VI* offers a fun collection of lists, followed by the *Appendixes—a surfing glossary* and a *global surf-o-dex* in *Part VII.*

Throughout the book, I have highlighted certain key infor-
mation with the icon above. Each of these tidbits points out a particularly kooky act. Unless you have one of those freaky photographic memories, there is no way you will remember everything in this book after a single reading. Hopefully some of the information comes flooding back when you go surfing. Better yet, take it to the beach with you. Between sessions, you can look up any problems you might be having and figure out how to correct them. Maybe the next edition will be laminated so you can take it into the water. Until then, good luck and happy surfing.

PART I: BASIC SURFOLOGY

CHAPTER 1 – WHAT IS SURFING?

In This Chapter
Surfing Defined (Sort Of)
Surf Story
What a Rush!
Surfing for Fitness
Surfing as Therapy
Surfing as Religion
Surfing Lifestyle
Surfing Careers
Surfing as a Sport
*Warning—Close This Book
    Immediately . . . or Else

PART 1: BASIC SURFOLOGY

CHAPTER 1 – WHAT IS SURFING?

Before delving into the many facets of surfing, let me get one thing off my chest. Riding waves represents something different to each person who does it, and those various perspectives are part of what makes surfing so interesting. But there is one thing I cannot accept. Clicking a television remote control or a computer mouse ain't surfing! These idle pursuits could not be any further removed from the topic at hand. Nor does the practice of taking advantage of your friends' generosity by camping on their love-seat bear any relation to riding waves. These acts have nothing in common with surfing, and to describe them as such constitutes a sort of blasphemy. So, if you insist on perpetuating the terms "channel surfing," "surfing the net," and "couch surfing," you are, and always will be, a kook. Now that you know what surfing isn't, let's discuss what it is.

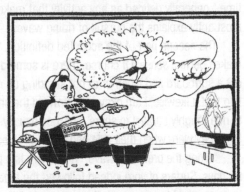

FOR THE RECORD, THIS GUY IS NOT SURFING.

Surfing Defined (Sort Of)

Most definitions of surfing run something like this: "The sport of riding atop a surfboard toward the shore along the crest of a wave." That explanation misses the mark on several counts. The first issue is whether or not surfing is a sport. Physical activity, the principle facet of any sport, is highly prevalent with surfing. Sports, on the other hand, invariably include a set of rules, and this is where things get fuzzy. Sure, competitive surfing, with its rulebook, exists and has grown leaps and bounds in a relatively short time. However, for the overwhelming majority of surfers, the only rules that apply are the laws of physics (except for some particularly acrobatic young surfers who routinely challenge the law of gravity). We have no time limits, no scoring system, no boundaries, and no referee. And despite the efforts of some within the surfing industry, we are unlikely to ever see surfers vying for an Olympic gold alongside every activity that even remotely resembles a sport.

So, if not a sport, can surfing be explained as an act, an occupation, or maybe an art form? Arguably, it could pass for any of those. Considering how easily several hours can fly by while you are surfing, perhaps "pastime," generally defined as any activity that makes time pass pleasantly, most aptly explains the pursuit of riding waves.

The second part of the accepted definition, "riding atop a surfboard," makes perfect sense. Of course, there is some debate over what is or is not a surfboard and whether or not standing up matters, but we will not get into that. Likewise, I am okay with "toward the shore." Most surfers tend to ride roughly parallel to shore, but they usually finish closer to the beach than they were when their ride began. No problems there.

"Along the crest of a wave," now there is a phrase that has seen better days. Surfers of yore indeed followed the tapering, top part of a wave to its eventual terminus with the single-mindedness of a coonhound tailing a pesky varmint. Through the middle part of the twentieth century, riding "along the crest of a wave" represented nothing less than the ultimate in surfing performance. A few generations back, that all changed as surfers began exploring a wave's every nook and cranny rather than stoically hitching a ride. For those who are just getting the hang of it or who are physically unable to turn, "along the crest" remains the name of the game. For everyone else, the notion of zigzagging one's personal signature along a wave continues to take surfing further away from its unswerving past. Meanwhile, slotting oneself inside the hollow, churning innards of a wave, or "getting tubed," ranks on the top of most any surfer's list of favorite things. After experiencing the unequivocal thrill of riding inside the curl, everything else pales in comparison.

Finally, the time spent actually "riding" makes up a miniscule portion of the time attributed to surfing. Before any riding can take place, one must check the conditions, suit up and wax up, paddle out, get in line, choose a wave, and catch it. The ride typically measures in seconds, and after that another hunk of time—typically anywhere from a few minutes to half an hour—will pass before the next wave is ridden. In the interim, there is more paddling, and often sitting, waiting, searching, and hoping. That being said, the standard definition falls miserably to explain surfing. It would take a whole book to do that, which is precisely the reason we are here.

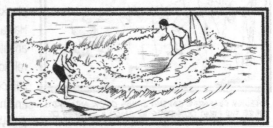

THE TWO MAIN METHODS OF SURFING ARE LONGBOARD-ING AND SHORTBOARDING.

Surf Story

Right about the time Jesus allegedly strutted across a lake, some dudes in the South Pacific took the miracle out of walking on water. No one knows for sure when man first stood atop a board and rode a wave toward the shore, but the event likely happened over two thousand years ago either in Peru or one of the islands near Tahiti.

These cultures were dependent upon the ocean for their survival and navigated in and out of the surf regularly. Sooner or later, a fisherman was bound to stroke his canoe into a wave on the way in from work and stand up to get a better view of the ride. Seeing how much fun he was having, some kids along the shoreline likely snatched up the canoe and headed

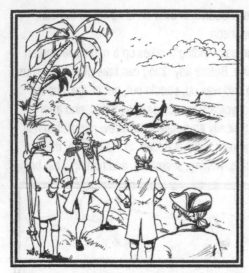

ENGLISH SEAFARER CAPTAIN JAMES COOK AND CREW WERE THE FIRST OUTSIDERS TO CATCH A GLIMPSE OF SURFING IN HAWAII.

out for some fun. As a result, surfing was born.

As Polynesians migrated to Hawaii, they found these reef-encircled volcanic islands perfectly suited for cultivating the pursuit of riding waves. Using solid wooden planks as long as 18 feet, Hawaiians made surfing an integral part of their religion and culture. British sea captain James Cook and his crew became the first Westerners to behold surfing during a 1777 visit to Tahiti. Of one particularly adept waverider, Cook wrote, "I could not help concluding that this man felt the most supreme pleasure while he was driven on so fast and so smoothly by the sea." As Cook sailed into Hawaii's Kealakekua Bay a few months later, he found that surfers were more common in these parts than nerds at a *Star Trek* convention.

Tragically, Western diseases decimated the Hawaiian population within a century of Cook's arrival, and the scant survivors were coerced into abandoning the surfing life. Puritanical missionaries visiting Hawaii in the 1800s frowned not only on the frivolity of surfing, but also its skimpy attire and inherent intermingling of the sexes. By the end of the nineteenth century, surfing was practically dead to the world.

Riding waves owes its eventual rebirth to a few individuals who spread the word that surfing was worthy of saving. Author Jack London cruised his boat into Hawaii in 1907 and plunked himself on the sand at Waikiki. There, he met a globetrotting journalist named Alexander Hume Ford who coaxed the visitor into a surf lesson. London took a beating, but he loved it. He extolled the virtues of this "royal sport for the natural kings of the earth" In a

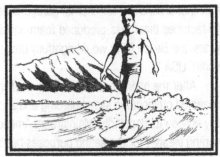

ASIDE FROM BEING AN OLYMPIC CHAMPION SWIM-MER AND HOLLYWOOD ACTOR, HAWAIIAN DUKE KAHANAMOKU (1890-1968) RANKS AS THE FATHER OF MODERN SURFING.

national magazine article, as well as in a book depicting his travels.

Surfing's own version of Johnny Appleseed, Duke Kahanamoku, soon emerged from along this same stretch of sand to spread the word internationally. In the 1912 Olympics in Stockholm, Duke became a national hero by claiming gold for the United States in the 100-meter freestyle. As comfortable as Duke was in the pool, his true home was the ocean, and in the years that followed he introduced his beloved pastime to the rest of the world. Kahanamoku's regal presence and global ambassadorship earned him a reputation as the Father of Modern Surfing. The first two world wars, along with limited and cumbersome equipment, kept the wave riding population in check for several decades, but a boom was coming.

If Duke was surfing's father, then its mother, it could be said, was a giggly, unsuspecting teenager from Brentwood, California. In the summer of '56, fifteen-year-old Kathy Kohner spent her vacation learning to surf from the guys at Malibu. Being a girl and something of a midget, she was dubbed "Gidget." Kohner relayed her surf stories to her father Frederick, who turned them into a best-selling novel. Once Hollywood got its hands on Gidget in 1959, surfing exploded into a national phenomenon. It didn't hurt that around the same time, garage-built wooden boards were replaced by factories that mass-produced foam-and-fiberglass boards. Within a few years, the Beach Boys would rightfully proclaim, "Everybody's gone surfin', surfin' USA."

After the boom, boards became smaller and sleeker, and surfing spawned offshoots in skateboarding and snowboarding that would eventually eclipse its popularity. Mainstream America has since embraced the surfing lifestyle for marketing purposes but still fails to recognize it as much more than a pleasurable diversion.

What a Rush!

Upon catching his first wave at Waikiki, Jack London declared feeling "ecstatic bliss" at rushing through the ocean at such a rapid clip. Unfortunately, a wicked sunburn kept him from returning to the beach the following day to learn how to stand up, but his experience was nonetheless breathtaking.

That rush of adrenaline is surfing's hook. The sensation is what snatches newbie waveriders from the "unjazzed" and instills in them an insatiable addiction for more. "Only a surfer," one saying goes, "knows the feeling."

I could fill this entire volume trying to explain "The Feeling" and still fall flat. Short of physically taking you to the beach and pushing you into a wave, any description will prove incomplete. Can surfing be compared to shooting down a waterslide? Not really, considering a waterslide is man-made, prefabricated fun, and thus incomparable. What about snowboarding? It takes place on a natural surface, but the surface of a mountain, unless you're riding an avalanche, isn't moving like a wave. Bungee jumping? Perhaps the sensation of weightlessness is similar, but you know in the back of your mind that the cord will save you. The best comparison might be flying. Not flying in an airplane, but rather Superman-style. Humans cannot fly, but you can at least imagine what it might feel like.

The feeling is present on wave one, as it was with London, and it's still there after a lifetime in the water. Initially, simply catching a wave is enough to capture the feeling, but sooner or later even something as majestic as riding waves can become humdrum. Fortunately, with each new skill learned, the feeling returns. Standing up offers a thrill, followed by angling parallel to the wave and riding it all the way to the sand. Eventually, acquiring that feeling requires catching a bigger or steeper wave, or perhaps pulling off a new maneuver. On the other hand, a new challenge can be as simple as trying out a different type of surfboard or traveling to a different place to surf. The beauty is that no matter how long someone surfs or how proficient one becomes, there is always something new to learn. The feeling can last forever.

Surfing for Fitness

Experienced surfers appear to exert minimal effort during a session. They stroke through the water as if powered by a motor, barely move their arms when picking off a wave, and seem to beam themselves all over the water by simply leaning one way or the other. Don't let them fool you. Surfing requires massive amounts of energy, especially in the beginning.

In the beginning, all the rigmarole involved in catching a few waves can seem like work, not to mention the ample opportunities for embarrassment, bodily harm, and ingesting gallons of seawater. But do not lose sight of the reward, those few seconds of slipping into Superman's boots and soaring above Metropolis without a safety net. For the fleeting instant of joy, the work is worth it.

There is a flip side to surfing's physically demanding nature. Once one grows accustomed to all the paddling and pushing up and gains some sense of proficiency, the pain disappears. All that remains is the fun. After a month or so of surfing, you forget that you're even exercising. You are, of course, and the subsequent physical benefits are numerous. Find an avid surfer, and what you will have is one physically fit human being. Weight loss, muscle tone, and improved stamina go hand-in-hand with riding waves. Surfing burns calories away like nobody's business. Nothing rouses an appetite like a few hours in the water. As a result, many a post-session meal rivals that of an NFL player's post-game chow-down.

Fitness is not a bad reason to take to the water, far better than, say, learning to surf in order to impress a potential mate or because you think you'd look totally cool cruising along the strip with a board strapped to the roof. Surfing, after all, provides far more enjoyment and variety than spin class. And you do not need to make an appointment or pay any dues. Just show up and paddle out. Your session can last anywhere from half an hour to all day if you have the energy. The longer you surf, the more physical benefits you will receive.

Surfing as Therapy

Perhaps the greatest impact surfing can have on an individual is therapeutic. Hydrotherapy, or the use of water for soothing pains and treating diseases, dates back to ancient Asian cultures. While no studies have been conducted regarding the healing powers of riding waves, most any surfer will contend that there is nothing a good day of surfing won't cure.

Surfing does not so much allow its participants to forget about their problems as much as it requires them to do so. Complete focus is a prerequisite to riding a wave. A lack of focus often leads to disaster. But more than that, an old maxim warns, "Never turn your back on the ocean," and for good reason. Ignore the surf, and eventually it will make you pay.

The required attention to detail, rather than having a draining effect on surfers, provides just the opposite. They return to land utterly refreshed, ready to tackle any obstacle that comes their way. Living in the moment has long been a tenet of Zen philosophy, and this way of thinking provides clear advantages.

Perhaps Miki Dora, surfing's iconoclastic Dark Knight of yore, best explained how surfing's therapeutic benefits extend beyond boundaries. "My whole life is escape," Dora raved in the 1990 *Film Surfers: The Movie.* "My whole life is this wave. I drop into 'em, set the whole thing up, pull up the bottom turn, pull up into it and shoot for my life, going for broke, man . . . and behind me all the shit goes over my back—the screaming parents, teachers, police, priests, politicians, kneeboarders, windsurfers. They're all going over the falls headfirst into the (bleep)ing reef and I'm shooting for my life and when it starts to close out I pull out through the bottom or out the back . . . and I pick up another one and do the same goddamn thing."

Surfing as Religion

Subscribe to it or not, surfing is a religion. Think about it. What is common among all of the world's religions? First, a set of beliefs or practices. Surfers believe that waves are for riding, and they practice their ideas

not just on Sunday mornings, but whenever the Supreme Being—Mother Nature or the Wave God Huey—sees fit to send some surf. The practice includes customs and rituals—among them praying for and making sacrifices for waves and gathering at surf movies. It has constructed houses of worship—surf shops. It can bring about

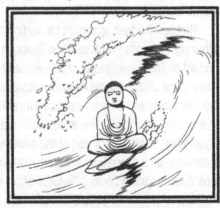

OF COURSE THE BUDDHA SURFED! HOW ELSE COULD HE HAVE BECOME SO ENLIGHTENED?

spiritual awakening and inspire practitioners to take up charitable causes such as environmental conservation. It teaches us about life. It leads many to abandon their previous routines and reconstruct their entire ways of living—their friends, their jobs—around riding waves. For untold numbers of surfers, it provides nothing less than salvation.

Surfing's connection with religion is nothing new. In pre-contact Hawaii, surfing was so much a part of the culture that it took on religious significance. Nowadays anyone can throw a credit card on the counter and walk out of a surf shop with a fresh surfboard, but in the Islands a new stick required some sacrifice. Kahunas, ancient Hawaiian priests, offered prayers and placed an offering of dead fish at the base of a tree that would be chopped down and carved into a board.

The late Tom Blake, architect of the surfboard fin and the hollow board in the 1930s, is considered one of surfing's holy men. Blake first delved into the religious elements of surfing with his controversial 1969 *Surfing* magazine article, "Voice of the Wave." He later carved his most famous mantra, "Nature=God," into a boulder in his native Wisconsin. Needless to say, he was a believer.

Perhaps the best argument for surfing as a religion comes from University of Florida Professor Bron Taylor. In addition to his work as editor-in-chief of *The Encyclopedia of Religion and Nature*, Taylor penned a 2007 essay in the *Journal of the American Academy of Religion* entitled "Surfing into Spirituality and a New, Aquatic Nature Religion." In the lengthy article, he exercises a scholarly lens to establish wave riding as a legitimate creed, arguing that "a significant part of the evolving global, surfing world can be understood as a new religious movement in which sensual experiences constitute its sacred center." Taylor is either correct in his theory, or he has provided an excuse for people to ditch work and go surfing. One way or the other, I applaud his efforts.

Surfing Lifestyle

Surfing as a way of life owes its creation to a fateful 1920 meeting in a theater lobby in Detroit. Duke Kahanamoku, already a national hero for his swimming exploits, stopped in with some Olympic teammates on their way across the country to watch a newsreel of themselves from the recent games in Belgium. Duke was approached by many admirers, one of them Tom Blake, then a parentless eighteen-year-old kid who longed to escape the cold, boring Midwest. They shook hands, and the youngster "felt that somehow he had included an invitation to me to come over to his own Hawaiian Islands." Blake jumped at the imaginary offer and went on to cultivate the nomadic, carefree lifestyle that would become synonymous with surfing.

Over the next couple decades, Blake learned to surf, revitalized several ancient Hawaiian ideas, revolutionized surfboards and surf rescue, wrote the first book on surfing (*Hawaiian Surfriders*, 1935), invented the waterproof camera housing, and established the lifestyle that surfers lead today. He was smitten by the quiet, simple Hawaiian way of life, and in his subsequent travels around the mainland he "promoted" the surfing lifestyle. The hallmarks of Blake's existence included a healthy diet, ample physical activity in the water, casual dress, and the freedom to roam.

Mainstream America got its first dose of this way of life with Gidget's cavorting at Malibu, leading to a nationwide craze that has since intensified. The "it's all good" attitude emerged as a beachy teenager mentality, but it is no longer bound by age or geography. Surfing as a marketing gimmick is used to sell everything from credit cards to medications for erectile dysfunction. Surf culture is rooted in the love of the ocean, but it has expanded to include music, fashion, lingo, literature, and movies. The unfortunate part is that most of the people who buy into the lifestyle with their pocketbooks will never ride a wave. In other words, they have purchased an idea instead of an experience.

Surfing Careers

While the growth of the surf industry hardly rates a mention alongside the explosion of the computer industry during the same period of time, the business of surfing has expanded dramatically, even exponentially, in the last half-century. Some people may still be surprised to learn that a surf industry exists at all, and that some of the higher profile companies are traded on the New York Stock Exchange. In fact, surfing is a multibillion-dollar enterprise that extends far past the mom-and-pop surf shops nestled away in tiny beach communities.

The opportunities for careers in and around surfing have likewise expanded. Whereas the only occupation associated with riding waves was once "surfboard builder," nowadays the list is extensive. Retail surf shops entered the picture as a potential career choice not long after the demand for mass-produced boards in the late '50s and early '60s. Surf apparel followed, and nowadays these companies employ entire teams of designers, artists, marketers, and salespeople. Surf media has also grown, providing opportunities in journalism, photography, video, and web design. Other employment opportunities include surf schools, surf travel, and wave forecasting. And while many of these positions cannot compete monetarily with other industries, the deficits are more than made up for in fringe

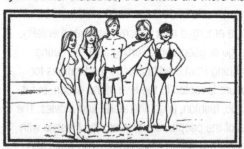

A CAREER AS A PROFESSIONAL SURFER
BRINGS ALONG MANY PERKS.

benefits. For a surfer, the chance to continue living the lifestyle at work is priceless.

No career in surfing, or in any other industry for that matter, could possibly equal the life of a professional surfer. These guys and gals get paid, some of them quite handsomely, to travel to exotic locations around the world and do what they love to do. They would be surfing whether someone paid them to or not, so the idea of making a living from it is icing on the cake. Other than the occasional flight delay, sunburn, or deranged groupie, life doesn't get any better than this.

Surfing as a Sport

For any definition of surfing, "sport" far from covers all the bases. As you've just learned, surfing is more than a game. On the other hand, the sporting aspect is precisely the point for some surfers, and not merely the pros. Many amateur wave riders, young and old alike, dedicate themselves to competition. These combatants gladly cough up their entry fees and spend their weekends in an ongoing pursuit of trophies and bragging rights. They do not represent a large percentage of all surfers, but their presence in the lineup is unmistakable. Their aggressive and competitive nature can turn any session into a wave-catching scrum. We will address the ins and outs of competition in a later chapter, so right now suffice it to say that some people indeed look at surfing as a sport.

Warning—Close This Book Immediately . . . or Else

If you are perfectly content with your life as it is, and you are considering taking up surfing, please don't. The greatest danger lies not in any physical harm you might incur in the water but in the addictive nature of riding waves. There is a distinct possibility that you will get hooked on surfing. When that happens, your life will be turned upside down with all the intensity of a two-story Pipeline bone-crusher detonating on the razor-sharp reef.

Here is how it works: You successfully ride a few waves; you want more; at school or work you lose focus on the task at hand and start doodling waves on notebooks and memo pads; driving down the street you stick your arm out the window and "surf" the oncoming rush of air with your hand; the ocean awakens from a month-long flat spell just as an important prior engagement nears; you blow off your responsibilities because the surf forecast calls for the waves to be gone by tomorrow; to help you forget about your now crumbling life, you go surfing; and the cycle repeats.

Then again, you may find surfing to be just awful. The water may be too cold. A crab may pinch your toe on your way into the ocean. Another surfer may berate you for paddling for "his" wave. A wipeout may result in a board to the head and a nasty gash requiring stitches. A parking ticket may be waiting for you back at your car.

All of those things and more have happened to me throughout the years, but none of them have discouraged me from surfing. For me, it's too late. I'm a lost cause. But for you there is still hope. This is your last chance to get away while you still can. I hope you make the right decision.

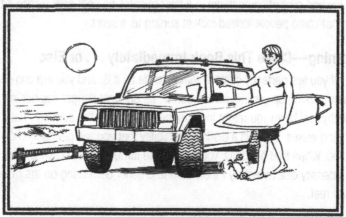

PINCHED TOES AND PARKING TICKETS ARE MINOR INCONVENIENCES THAT
COME ALONG WITH SURFING.

PART I: BASIC SURFOLOGY

CHAPTER 2 - READY, SET . . . SURF

In This Chapter

Since you are reading this chapter, you have probably never surfed, at least not with a whole lot of success. Therefore, you are still under the impression that there are things in life other than surfing that actually mean something. Savor these final moments as a landlubber. Pretty soon, it'll all be a distant memory—the boring old hobbies, the comatose weekends camped in front of the telly, even the love handles.

You're about to learn the basic steps that will enable you to partake in the Royal Hawaiian Pastime. Next thing you know, you will be praying for hurricanes, dripping salt water from your nose at the dinner table, and finally understanding what all the fuss is about.

From the Car to the Shore

The often-overlooked portion of the surfing experience known as "getting to the beach" deserves at least a mention. I realize you're antsy to get in the water, but there are a few details that warrant your consideration.

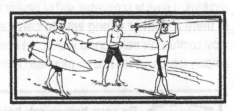

WHILE YOU CAN CARRY YOUR SURFBOARD IN ANY MANNER YOU WISH, THESE GUYS DEMONSTRATE SOME OF THE MORE ACCEPTED METHODS.

Where will you park? – Maybe there is free parking, but probably not. Bring money for a pay lot and plenty of change if there are parking meters. Obviously, the closer you can get to the beach the better. Check any nearby signs for additional information. There may be a certain time that parking is prohibited, such as certain mornings for street sweeping. There are better ways of spending money than parking tickets.

How will you get dressed? – If you drive to the beach in your bathing suit or wetsuit, getting suited up isn't an issue. However, if you need to change, is there a bathroom nearby, or do you have a towel you can wrap around you?

Some places might not allow changing in public. And when you are finished surfing, will you drive home sopping wet and drip all over your car's interior?

What about your keys? – If you do not have someone with you who will be staying on the beach, you need to stash your keys somewhere. Many boardshorts and wetsuits have a place for a key, so you might be able to take it with you. Consider a Hide-A-Key for stowing it somewhere on your vehicle. Or, you can hide the key in the bumper or in the coils above the wheels. Look around and make sure no one is watching. Some surfers utilize a smooth, "Oops, I dropped my wax, better bend down to pick it up" move to inconspicuously slip the key into its hiding place.

Should you leave anything on the beach? – Belongings are usually safer locked in the car. However, at some spots the locals won't hesitate to bust out a window to see what valuables are sitting inside. If you are somewhere that seems dubious, leave nothing in the vehicle and roll down the windows. It pays to know what sort of environment you are dealing with.

Is there a right or wrong way to carry a board? – However you are most comfortable transporting your board from the car to the shore is fine. A heavy longboard can rest on your head with one hand on each side for

---

"HEY, KOOK!" **Do your homework before pulling up to a new spot.** If you have never been to a particular beach, find out what kind of place it is before pulling up to go surfing. Generally, you will not have a problem. However, at some spots, the locals do not take kindly to strangers. Be careful where you park and what you leave in your vehicle. If the place you are going surfing has a reputation for territorial locals, do not show up unless you know someone. And do not pull up at a crowded spot with a carload of visiting newbie surfers.

balance. Otherwise, most surfers carry their board nose-first with the deck facing out. There is no real reason for this other than perhaps preventing the wax from smearing all over you.

Surf-Ups

You know how to swim, right? Thank goodness, because it would have been back to the pool for you, buddy. The ocean, with its unpredictability, is nowhere to learn how to swim. Since you're a veritable Michael Phelps, the next step is the "surf-up." Like the name implies, a surf-up is much like a push-up. The only difference is, instead of just pushing up and going back down, you will thrust upward into a standing position.

First, find a flat area of sand and do not worry about embarrassing yourself in front of fellow beachgoers. (If you're overly self-conscious, practice at home on the floor.) These dry runs allow you to work out any kinks without the consequences you'll encounter in the water.

Lay flat, and try to imagine a wave approaching you from behind. Begin paddling one arm at a time, making certain your head is up and your hands are cupped like two little ice cream scoopers. After several strokes, place your hands just below your shoulders as with a push-up. Next, in one (hopefully) smooth motion, pop your body up and bring your feet underneath you, planting them firmly one in front of the other. Your hands should act as stabilizers at this point, keeping the board steady until your feet are planted. Many beginners, in their hurry to stand, release their grip too early. As a result, their feet usually end up in the wrong place and their ride ends before it truly begins.

Are you regular or goofy? A regularfoot, also known as a naturalfoot, surfs with left foot forward, while a goofy-foot stands with the right foot in front. In the early days most surfers rode with their left foot forward, which is why the other way became "goofy." Nowadays, there's nothing goofy about a goofyfoot. Both sides are equally represented. To determine your stance,

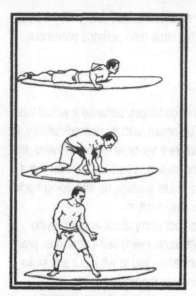

GET COMFORTABLE PERFORMING THE "SURF-UP" IN ONE FLUID MOTION BEFORE ENTERING THE WATER.

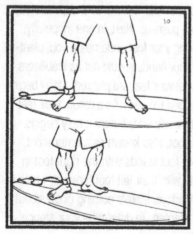

it doesn't really matter if you're left or right-handed. Try both stances and settle on whichever feels more comfortable. If you aren't sure, stand with your feet side-by-side and have someone push you in the chest. One of your feet will instinctively drop back for support. Whichever way you are standing, that is your surfing stance.

Your feet should be roughly parallel at just over shoulders' width apart. Instead of pointing your feet forward toward the nose, they must be angled at a bearing of around two o'clock for a regular-foot and ten o'clock if you're goofy. Plant your feet flat on the deck of the board for maximum support. Bend your knees slightly in order to absorb any bumps during the ride. The lower your center of gravity is, the better. Standing straight up is a no-no. Once you get your feet in place, for goodness sakes, look where you are going!

Practice several surf-ups before entering the water. Check

THE DIFFERENCE BETWEEN SUCCESS AND FAILURE OFTEN COMES DOWN TO CORRECT (TOP) AND INCORRECT (BOTTOM) FOOT POSITIONING.

your stance in a mirror to see if you're doing it correctly. It is okay to start out slow and increase your speed once you get the hang of it. If you are having trouble popping up, try sliding your back foot forward as you're pushing up. This will give you better leverage and your back leg will already be in position. Having an experienced surf instructor proves extremely valuable if you're having trouble getting to your feet. There is likely an easy solution, but you may have trouble figuring it out on your own.

"HEY, KOOK!" **Keep your hands planted.** When practicing your surf-ups, keep your hands on the sides of the board until you get your feet in place. Many beginners let go too early and try to get up using only their legs. This mistake puts undue pressure on the legs and makes standing far more difficult than it needs to be. Your arms will act as support beams that keep the board steady until you are up and riding.

Before Entering the Water

Know your equipment and, most importantly, know the surf conditions. These basic requirements, routinely overlooked by beginners, can prevent a world of trouble. Neither takes more than a few minutes, and the first part can be accomplished at home prior to hitting the beach.

Make sure your board is ready for action. See that it doesn't have any dings, or open wounds that may take on water or potentially cause injury. If you plan on keeping your board for a while, any holes or cracks should be repaired immediately. (See "Caring for Your Stick" in Chapter 10.) If your board has removable fins, confirm that they are securely screwed into place. The same routine goes for a rental board; check it out thoroughly before leaving the shop.

Don't show up at the beach without the two most crucial accessories for your board—a leash and some wax. Check to see that your leash is firmly fastened to the board, and give your wax-job a quick touchup. (See "Wax" in Chapter 11.) Many rentals are softboards that have a textured surface and don't need to be waxed. If you are unsure, ask someone.

Now that you are properly equipped, take some time to survey the surf. (This is a great opportunity to do a bit of stretching as you scope out the sea. See "Stretching" in Chapter Six.) Watch as other surfers enter the water. There may be a path of least resistance that can offer an easy paddle into the lineup as opposed to a nightmarish beating. This is where rip currents (see "Currents" in Chapter Five) can offer a free ride.

Study the surfers in the water as they wait for waves. Try to determine if they are drifting one way or the other. This is how you check for evidence of any cross-shore current, a potentially dangerous element that must be accounted for.

Once you have spotted the waves you plan to surf, find a marker on land that lines up with your ideal takeoff spot. Your marker could be a lifeguard stand, umbrella, sand dune, beach house, hotel, or any other structure that isn't moving. (Later, you'll want to glance shoreward every few minutes to make sure you haven't drifted from your original takeoff spot. If you've moved, paddle back to your marker or return to the beach and walk to it before paddling back out.)

"HEY, KOOK!" **Use The Buddy System.** Go surfing with a friend. There are plenty of other kooks out there. Not only is it advisable to always enter the ocean with a partner for safety reasons, the camaraderie that forms among fellow surfers builds a special bond. Knowing that someone is keeping an eye out for you, not to mention offering the occasion hoot of encouragement, can provide a boost of confidence.

Pre-Surf Checklist

Before paddling out, account for each of the following items. By doing so, you will avoid many potential accidents and ensure a safe and enjoyable session. In the beginning, this may take some time, but it is worth the trouble. Gradually the answers to these questions will come more quickly.

Wind – What direction is it blowing? How is this affecting the surf?

Tide – Is it coming in or going out? The surf can change dramatically due to tidal fluctuations.

Currents – Is there a potentially dangerous longshore or rip current flowing through the lineup?

Hazards – Are there any obstructions in the lineup that might have to be dealt with while paddling or surfing?

Entry and exit – Where is the easiest and safest place to paddle out and return to shore?

Takeoff Spot – Where is the best place to set up shop in the lineup in order to catch waves?

Consistency – How often are waves coming in? Are there long lulls or is the surf pouring through continuously?

How it's Breaking – Are the waves big or small, fast or slow, steep or sloping?

Crowd – How many people are surfing? Will I be alone? Will one more person be one too many?

Local Regulations – During summer, surfing may be "black-balled" during certain times of the day. Check with a lifeguard or local authority if you're unsure. Some localities issue citations not only for surfing, but also for surfing too close to a pier or other structure and for surfing without a leash.

"HEY, KOOK!" **Put your leash on the right way.** Fasten your leash around the ankle of your back leg. If you are a regular-foot, that means you wear your leash on the right leg, and if you are a goofyfoot it goes on the left leg. Secure the Velcro band low and tight around the ankle. Once fastened, see that the band is turned so that the cord emerges from the back rather than the front. That way you are less likely to trip over it while trying to stand up.

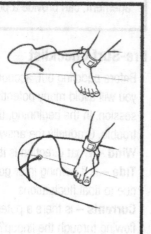

The Lay of the Land

Football fields, baseball diamonds, and curling sheets are each divided into distinct areas with fancy names. Surf spots are not as delineated, but they have various zones that possess distinct characteristics. Just as you would not go curling without knowing the "hog lines" for the "button," you shouldn't surf without an understanding of the playing field. **The key areas are as follows:**

Shoreline – where the beach meets the ocean

Shorebreak – generally steep waves that break directly onto the shoreline or just beyond it; fast-breaking waves that are not easily ridden

Trench – deep, waveless area usually located between the shorebreak and the lineup

Channel – deep, waveless passage perpendicular to the shoreline used for paddling out

Lineup – can include the entire surfing zone; also refers to the area at the outer edge of the sandbar or reef, where surfers sit to await approaching waves

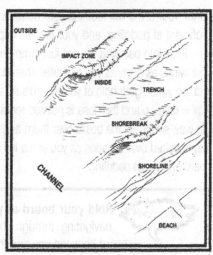

TO A BIRD, THIS IS WHAT A TYPICAL SURFING LINEUP LOOKS LIKE.

Impact zone – area in which the waves initially break; not a smart place to hang out unless you are a water photographer

Inside – part of the lineup that is closest to shore; usually a shallower area with smaller waves than the main takeoff spot, "farther inside" indicates an area closer to shore

Outside – outermost area of the lineup, "farther outside" means a greater distance from the beach

Paddling Makes the World Go 'Round

This is the part of surfing that you don't see in the travel brochures. Paddling makes surfing possible, but nobody likes it. At the outset of your surfing life, you will regard paddling with all the disdain of having a root canal. Your arms will feel like sore noodles for the first few days. Become proficient at paddling, and your life will improve dramatically.

Ease into paddling. Do not just jump on your board and start flapping your wings as soon as you hit water. There is an easier way. When walking into the water, grab hold of your board's rails, holding the board so that the wax is face up and the nose is pointed forward. If you encounter waves along the way, simply lift the board over them and lunge forward to keep from getting knocked over. As soon as you see a lull in the wave action, get on the board and begin paddling.

"HEY, KOOK!" **Hold your board at your side.** When it comes to navigating through the shorebreak, carrying your board between you and the surf is an invitation for disaster. A breaking wave will potentially knock your board into you, hurling you backwards toward the shore. Likewise, do not stand between the wave and your board. In this instance, the board could be ripped from your hands and endanger another surfer. Holding the board at your side while maneuvering through the shore-break offers the safest and fastest route to the lineup.

Some paddling tips to remember:

Check your positioning – Your entire body should be centered on the surfboard. Crooked paddling is a no-no. You also do not want to be too far forward or too far back. If you are properly centered, your board will rest flat in the water with the nose slightly above it but not pointing skyward. A good rule of thumb is to position your body so that your toes are slightly hanging off the tail. Once you have found a state of equilibrium, you are in the "sweet spot."

Cup your hands – Cupped hands will help achieve maximum thrust with each stroke. There should be no space between your fingers.

Keep your eyes on the road – Your head should be up to see where you are going.

One arm at a time – Paddling should resemble freestyle swimming rather than the breaststroke. Reach deep towards the seafloor with each stroke. Concentrate on smooth, even strokes. This is no time for half effort.

Try knee paddling – When riding a longboard, knee paddling offers an alternative, whereby you paddle from a kneeling position with both arms moving in unison as opposed to alternating strokes. Balance will be an issue at first, but the extra elevation provides a better view of the surf. This approach also helps relieve a sore back. On the other hand, knee paddling was the reason the legs of so many surfers of the 1960s were covered with knobby growths known as surf knots.

Duck, Duck . . . Dive

Short of hearing the theme from *Jaws* while bobbing alone helplessly in the ocean, the most harrowing experience for a fledgling surfer is this: You hop on your board and begin paddling into an inviting sea. The sun is shining, the seagulls are singing, and you're thinking how happy you are to

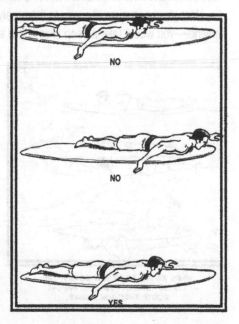

WHEN IT COMES TO PADDLING, DON'T BE TOO FAR BACK OR TOO FAR FORWARD.

be alive. Your confidence builds with each stroke until...what is that noise? You hear a faint rumbling that grows louder and louder. You catch a glimpse of the approaching wall of whitewater, yet there is a calm second of tranquility before the realization sets in. THAT WAVE IS GOING TO KILL ME!

Relax.

Easy for me to say, right? At this point, you have a few options. You can A) close your eyes, squeal like a baby pig, and pray that you will soon wake up snuggled in your warm, cozy bed; B) turn around to face the beach and hold on for the buckin' bronco ride of your life; or C) go under the wave.

Hopefully you didn't choose A. Option B isn't necessarily wrong and could be quite fun, but the best answer is C. Once you accept this fate, you must determine how to go about accomplishing such a feat.

Here you have more choices. In extremely large surf—say ten-foot Pipeline—you would take a deep breath and abandon ship just before impact, swimming as deep as possible to escape the turbulence. Expect a thorough rinse cycle before resurfacing. And always . . . I repeat, always, check to be sure no one is behind you before letting go of your surfboard.

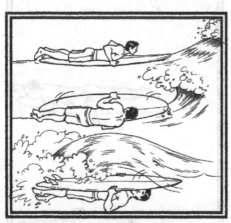

WHEN RIDING A LARGER BOARD, THE TURTLE TURN OFFERS THE SAFEST ROUTE THROUGH A WAVE.

Another alternative, one that longboarders and small kids tend to exercise due to the extreme buoyancy of their equipment, is the "Turtle Turn." This is where you paddle straight at the approaching wave, and just prior to contact, you and your board roll over as one. This requires a grip of steel to keep the board from being ripped from your hands. As soon as the wave passes, roll back over on top of your board and proceed.

Finally, we have our last alternative, the Duck Dive. I've never seen a turtle perform a turtle turn, but I am certain that ducks inspired the duck dive. This is the sleekest and least time-consuming method of penetrating an oncoming wave, therefore the most common. Because it requires you to temporarily sink your surfboard, the smaller the board, the easier it is to execute. Here is how it works:

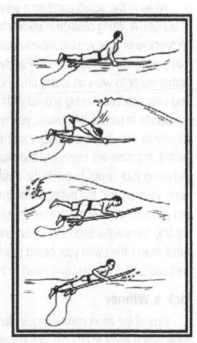

- When you see a breaking wave approaching, paddle directly toward it.
- At five to ten feet from impact, stop paddling and grab your board's rails approximately one-third of the way down from the nose. By applying downward pressure, you should be able to submerge the front half of your board just before the wave makes contact.
- As the wave goes over your head, apply pressure to the tail of your board using

THE DUCK DIVE PROVES AN INVALUABLE
TOOL THE BIGGER THE SURF GETS.

your knee or foot. This will sink the back half of your board, allowing the wave to travel over you without taking you with it.

- Your surfboard's buoyancy will return you to the surface after the wave has passed. Make sure you're centered and resume paddling.
- Repeat as necessary.
- Practice duck diving as much as possible on smaller days to prepare for when you will really need it. A good place to perfect this skill is in a pool. Duck diving skills will prove invaluable when the intensity of the surf increases.

Sit and Spin

While in the ocean awaiting a wave, surfers straddle their boards and sit upright. A sitting position is comfortable and allows the rider a better perspective of approaching waves. Balancing can be difficult at first, but with practice comes steadiness. Paddle beyond the breaking waves into calmer water to work on sitting up. Once you are able to sit without tipping over, practice turning around with your board from this position. When you decide to paddle for a wave, you will need to spin somewhat quickly. In order to spin, first scoot back toward the tail of the board. By moving to the tail, the nose will rise out of the water. Then, rotate by kicking your feet and using your hands to guide the board in the direction you're turning. The faster you can spin the better. Sometimes a wave pops up unexpectedly and you will not have much time if you hope to catch it. Once your board is pointing toward the beach, lie down and start paddling for the wave. Initially, rather than sitting with your board pointed out to sea, try sitting parallel to the beach. That way you only need to turn 90 degrees rather than 180.

Pick a Winner

One of the most common questions from a new surfer is, "How do I know which wave to catch?" Unfortunately, there's no simple answer. Wave knowledge is like seamanship; experience is the only true teacher. Who's going to learn more: The person sitting in the classroom getting jammed full of information, or the one who spends the same time sailing the high seas? There are, however, a few guidelines that can help along the way.

Open your eyes – Study the surf conditions. Take note of where waves are breaking and where other people are catching them. Deciding where to sit in the lineup is difficult since there are usually no markers in the water. Conditions vary daily and even hourly as the tide changes, so you will need to keep attuned to the surf for the duration of your session. Sit approximately five yards beyond where the majority of waves are breaking to allow room to paddle and stand.

Quantity over quality – In the beginning, any wave you can catch is the right one. Riding the whitewater is encouraged during the initial stages in your development. Broken waves are much easier to pick up, and the repetition allows you to get accustomed to standing and riding. The more waves you catch—good or bad—the more ingrained the process of getting to your feet will become. You can get picky later.

Be a predator – Waves do not always come to you. Go to them. Paddle around the lineup and stalk your prey.

Pick up some scraps – Sometimes you will miss a wave and find yourself in perfect position to catch the next one. As soon as a wave passes without you, take a look over your shoulder at the next one before turning around and paddling back out.

Give the extra effort – When you think you have caught a wave, take a couple extra strokes to be certain. Many beginners will stand too early and lose the wave. You'll know you have it when you start dropping down the wave face.

Take a trial run – There is nothing wrong with taking at least one wave lying down. In fact, it is a great idea. Get used to the speed and try steering the board with your arms to get a feel for it.

Stand Up and Be Counted

Congratulations, you have caught a wave. You did not expect to be moving this rapidly, and in front of you the beach is getting closer by the second. It is time to evolve from lying on your board like a lump of primordial ooze into a standing modern man or woman, and fast. Are you ready?

"HEY, KOOK!" **Learn how NOT to nosedive.** Nosedives happen, but they are not fun. Augering in on takeoff is a surefire way to injure your body, your board, or both. Fortunately, there is usually a small window of opportunity once you see a nosedive coming. Nosedives occur when there is too much weight on the front of your board, so the solution is to shift that weight back as quickly as possible. To shift your weight, grab the rails as if to perform a duck dive and push your board out in front of you without letting go. Your legs will be hanging off the back as if on a kickboard. Lay on your belly for the elevator drop to the bottom of the wave. Once the turbulence subsides, you can pull yourself back into position and proceed with standing up.

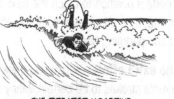

THE DREADED NOSEDIVE

If you catch several waves and cannot seem to find your footing, return to the beach for a few more practice runs. During each surf-up, watch your feet and make sure they are landing in the correct spots on the board. Remember, a wide stance lowers your center of gravity and makes things easier than a narrow one. Keep your knees bent and your back straight. Bending at the waist is a no-no. It gives you a "stink-butt" stance and throws you off balance. If you are tipping over in one direction each time you stand, it is probably a case of not putting your front foot in the center of the board. A few inches can make all the difference.

Bad habits are easy to come by. When it comes to standing up, these tendencies include improper hand placement when pushing up, getting on your knees, incorrect foot positioning, and a host of other problems. Things move quickly when you are learning to stand, so pinpointing the problem can prove difficult. If you are going it alone and having troubles, this is a good time to seek professional assistance.

Now What?

Remember the euphoria you felt on that first ride. You probably threw your arms skyward in elation and thought (or even yelled), "I'm surfing!" You are now hooked and yearning for more. For those not content to cruise in the whitewater, that excitement begins to wear off after a few dozen rides. Fortunately, you can get your groove back. The key is to tackle new challenges. With each accomplishment, the ecstasy returns.

The initial goal in surfing is to stand on your board while riding a wave. From there, the progression is pretty cut and dry. Not many people skip steps along the way. Here is what you can aspire to in the beginning:

Ride a wave to shore – "Beaching" a wave for the first time is a monumental achievement, usually prompting a leprechaun-ish leap for joy. Once you figure out where to put your feet and how to relax enough to absorb the occasional shock, you should be able to navigate the wave all the way to the sand. If you are lucky it could happen on your very first wave, or it could take anywhere from several rides to several days.

Catch a wave before it breaks – Whereas catching the whitewater propels you forward, getting into a wave early enables you to experience the thrill of dropping in. The more paddling practice you get, the quicker this will happen. It takes a bit of wave knowledge or a bit of luck, but either way you will not soon forget it.

Ride the line – Every wave either breaks to the left or right (judging from the water perspective rather than looking out from shore), and the next

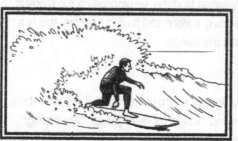

RIDING THE LINE PROVIDES THE FIRST STEP TOWARDS ADVANCED SURFING.

goal is to follow the breaking wave to its eventual end. When paddling for an unbroken wave, begin angling in the direction you wish to turn. Once you are up, apply pressure to that side of the board with your feet. Also turn your upper body slightly in that direction. Your board should start to turn, allowing you to set your course for a longer and more exciting ride.

Go backside – The natural inclination is to ride in the direction you are facing, which is to the right for a regular-foot and to the left for a goofyfoot. Slightly more difficult is riding in the opposite direction, since your back is to the wave. Surfing backside makes it harder to see what is going on with the wave. Strive to master riding backside. When you do, you open yourself to so many more waves.

Super-size me – The bigger the wave, the bigger the thrill. Seek out more challenging surf spots. Any rise in wave height brings a new adventure and a test of your skills. These milestones represent the tip of the learning iceberg. For a more extensive list of moves and tips on how to achieve them, see Part IV.

How Do I Stop This Thing?

World War II Japanese fighter pilots were trained to take flight. Safe landings were not necessary since these "kamikazes," as they were known, simply crashed into their targets. Needless to say, the surfing world does not need any kamikaze pilots. Before you take off on your first wave, try to imagine how you want it to end.

Depending on where you surf, a wave may or may not die out before reaching the shore. If your wave dissipates into deeper water, your ride will end of its own accord. Like it or not, you will stop. In this case, return to a prone position and paddle back out for another.

If the waves you are riding continue rolling to shore but you wish to make an exit, you have some options. One is the "eject" button. Jumping off your board is a quick way to abruptly end a ride. Before ejecting, consider the depth of the water beneath you as well as what lies at the bottom. You do not want to fillet your feet by leaping onto dry reef. If you are over a reef, landing flat offers the best chance for a safe exit. On the other hand, with several feet of water as a landing pad, a cannonball allows deeper penetration and less chance the wave will steamroll you. If you are riding down the line, diving over the back of the wave offers another escape. Just be sure you can get enough lift to clear the wave or else it will take you with it.

The "kick-out," of which there are several variations, provides another alternative, one that allows the rider and his surfboard to exit the wave together. Think of the kick-out as taking an off-ramp from the interstate. To perform a standard kick-out, simply lean in the direction where the wave offers the least resistance, and your board will follow. If you are on the shoulder of the wave, this will present no problems. If the wave is closing out, you will need to escape early or risk being sucked back over. Pulling through the wave itself is a trickier move. In larger surf, where the consequences of an unsuccessful kick-out are higher, this "standing island pullout" can be a lifesaver, but it takes practice. If you are too late to get out before the lip comes crashing down, or if you just want to head for the beach, simply straighten out (point your board toward the shore) and return to your belly by grabbing the rails and lowering yourself down.

As you have probably realized, you are not the only surfer around. There are other people in the lineup trying to ride some waves as well. Not only do you have to contend with the waves, now you must consider your fellow man. So, in the next chapter you will learn how to interact with other surfers without making a fool of yourself.

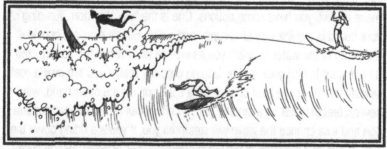

THREE FORMS OF KICK-OUTS – "THE FLY-AWAY" (LEFT), "THE STANDING ISLAND PULLOUT" (MIDDLE), AND THE STANDARD METHOD.

CHAPTER 3 - ETIQUETTE

In This Chapter

Manners are optional. During my semiannual round of golf, I often choose to ignore the unwritten code of the course. I think golf etiquette is silly. I would never do something that might injure another golfer, but as for whispering on the tee box and tiptoeing around the green so as not to violate someone's line of sight, phooey! With surfing, you can choose to follow established etiquette or not. The choice is yours. However, the consequences for breaking the rules in the lineup can be far greater than a sneer from some geezer in plaid pants. Since there is no official "marshall" in the water, or a referee to blow a whistle or throw a yellow flag, breaches of etiquette are handled by the surfers themselves by whatever means they see fit. Upon leaving the beach and entering the lineup, you are entering another world.

Surfing etiquette has been passed down through the ages, gaining importance as lineups become more crowded and subsequent dangers more common. The ocean is a beautiful place, but it can also be unpredictable and even deadly. Follow the rules, and your experience will be a more positive one. More than anything, kooks are guilty of breaking the basic code of surf etiquette. Since everything in this chapter explains how not be a kook, I have not highlighted anything with the "HEY, KOOK!" icon. All of it is critical.

Don't Drop In

At some surf spots, five surfers riding together on a single wave is the norm. With far more people in the water than there are waves to be ridden, some mayhem is inevitable. However, at anywhere

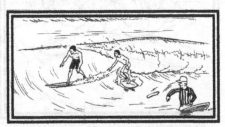

WHILE YOU MIGHT GET AWAY WITH IT, DROPPING IN ON ANOTHER SURFER IS NOT COOL.

other than at the most crowded of breaks, the general rule of thumb is "One man, one wave." (This rule is deceiving, because if the wave has a peak and peels off to the left and right, two surfers can ride without getting in each other's way.)

If you recall from "Now What?" in Chapter Two, one of the earliest objectives in surfing is to ride down-the-line, or parallel to the beach, as opposed to straight towards it. When two surfers ride in the same direction on a wave, it becomes the responsibility of the surfer in front to yield to the surfer in back. A "drop in," the most blatant violation of the surfing code, occurs when the surfer in front ignores this rule. Also known as "cutting off," "burning," or "snaking," this infringement of etiquette shows the utmost lack of respect. The surfer in back, so long as he is not behind the breaking part of the wave, has "inside position" and should be allowed to ride the wave unbothered.

There are exceptions. One surfer may have inside position, but also be sitting closer to shore. The surfer who is farther outside has the right of way even if he is in front of the other surfer.

Dropping in, aside from being rude, places both surfers at a heightened risk of injury. If one of the riders falls, his unmanned surfboard poses

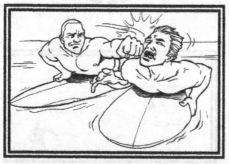

OCCASIONALLY, BEING A KOOK IS HARMFUL TO YOUR HEALTH.

an immediate danger to the other. Surfers can be a territorial and loyal bunch, and if you are seen dropping in on someone, you may be in for more than you bargained. At the least, the offending surfer is asking to be dropped in upon on the next wave. In some cases, a drop-in will earn a verbal or even physical retaliation. Snake someone at a localized surf spot, and the intrusion could result in the punching out of either your fins or your teeth.

Accidents will happen. You will, even if you are careful, eventually drop in on someone. Usually, a sincere apology will diffuse any potential situation. Communication helps avoid most run-ins.

Every time you see a wave that you want to catch, even before you take the first stroke, look around and make sure another surfer is not in a better position to catch it. There may already be someone riding the wave, so look down the line to see if the coast is clear. Skilled surfers are often able to navigate across waves that others consider closeouts, so never assume the other surfer is too far back to make a section. When in doubt, pull out. There will always be another wave.

Get Out of the Way

Nothing puts someone on the fast track to "kook-dom" quicker than getting in the way of another surfer. While no human should be so arrogant as to think he owns a particular wave, much less an entire swath of ocean, a surfer should be able to ride a wave without some uninformed bozo stumbling across his path. "Not getting the memo" is no excuse, because here it is: Get Out of the Way!

Not to overstate the obvious, but paddling into the path of someone who is riding a wave constitutes a major blunder. The offender not only ruins the ride for the other person, he increases his likelihood of getting run over. As an example, assume a surfer is riding down the line on a wave, and you are paddling out.

You have two choices:

1) Attempt to paddle faster than the surfer is traveling in order to make it over the shoulder, or unbroken part of the wave, or

2) Paddle in the opposite direction, even if it means you will get swamped by the whitewater. Easy decision, choose Option Two.

You will appreciate it when someone does the same for you.

Here's another situation. When you reach your destination in the lineup, look around. Is there someone sitting directly out to sea from where you are? If that person turns around to paddle for a wave, will he plow right into you? If an unexpectedly large wave breaks beyond that surfer, will he become a bowling ball and you a pin? If so, get out of the way! Most lineups allow ample space for everyone to spread out. Do not become a human bowling pin.

Finally, here is a simple word problem: Johnny is riding left on a wave. He is moving at ten miles per hour. You are riding the same wave heading right, also traveling at ten miles per hour. The two of you are on a collision course. Which surfer should assume the responsibility of avoiding the impending crash?

Need more time?

The answer is you, Stupid! Giving way ensures a safe exit and the opportunity to catch another wave. Any time you are riding toward another surfer and he at you, best to err on the side of safety.

The optimal means of staying out of the way is to surf spots that are not crowded. Until you become proficient at maneuvering among the waves and other surfers, you and a buddy should find your own little sandbar away from the pack. The waves may not be quite as good, but you will have a safer and more enjoyable session.

Navigating a Crowd

Sometimes there is no way around it; you either surf in a crowd or you don't get to surf. Not to worry. Diving into an already-congested lineup is not the end of the world. With some foresight, you might avoid getting run over. You could even make some new friends. Shoot, if you are really lucky, you may catch a wave.

As a beginner, exhaust all options before paddling into a crowd. Things move quickly in the lineup, especially when a wave is approaching. Novice surfers cannot move as swiftly as more experienced riders. In the heat of the

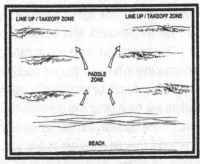

FOR AN EASY PADDLE AND PLENTY OF WAVES, EXAMINE THE LINEUP AND COME UP WITH A PLAN.

moment, you will feel like a sandlot quarterback thrown into an NFL game with a full-scale blitz coming.

Paddling out poses the initial challenge. Typically, one area of the lineup is packed while the surrounding regions aren't so bad. That congested spot is where the waves are focused. Do not, under any circumstances, attempt to paddle directly from the beach to this main peak. Instead, stay out of harm's way by paddling around the break. Sometimes waves are popping up all over, but there is usually a path of least resistance to one side or the other. Not only will you be doing everyone a favor, your trip to the lineup will be considerably easier.

The next task is the most difficult, being the one dude among many to end up in the perfect position to catch a wave. The lineup is not the deli counter, so do not expect to take a number and have it called in a few minutes. Every so often, dumb luck trumps preparation and a wave miraculously eludes everyone else in favor of the new guy. But like the total dork scoring the hottest babe, this generally only happens in movies. Being in the right place at the right time is an art form, honed through years of figuring out the nuances of a particular surf break. In the beginning, if you find yourself in what seems to be the ideal spot to catch a wave out of a crowded lineup, look again. Someone else is probably in better position. Be sure you double-check who is around you whenever paddling for a wave.

Communication in the lineup can help the wave-catching process run smoothly. Whenever you are paddling alongside another surfer for the same wave, do not be ashamed to ask which way he is going, left or right. Surfers ask each other this question regularly, and it shows respect on your part. On the flip side, you can let someone know you are heading in their direction if they do not seem to see you. A simple, "Hey, coming right," will suffice. Of course, if you happen to be an outsider at a localized spot, better to just keep your mouth shut and to wait for the next wave. If a wave

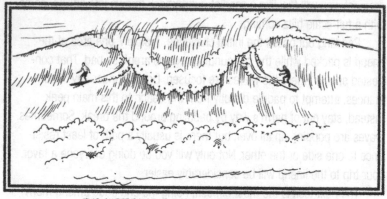

TWO SURFERS SPLIT A PEAK, AND EVERYONE'S HAPPY.

peels off in both directions, surfers will routinely "split the peak," one going right and the other left. Here again, communication is the key. "I'll go left" lets the other paddler know he can go right and everyone is happy.

When you finally get a wave to yourself, a crowded lineup becomes an obstacle course. In addition to reading the wave and struggling to make the most of this opportunity, there is invariably another surfer paddling directly into your chosen path. Do your best to avoid a collision. Since you have not learned to turn (that comes in Part IV), either jump off with enough space for your leash to stop the board or drop to your stomach and try to steer away from trouble. If you end up running over someone, just hope it is not an ornery local with an overabundance of testosterone.

Watch and Learn

There is an old story about a father and son looking down from a cliff at an empty bay filled with perfect waves. The son says to the father, "Dad, how about we run down the hill and catch one of those waves?" The father, in his eminent wisdom, responds, "Son, let's walk down the hill and catch all of them." Okay, so the real story involves bulls and cows and birds and bees, but you get the picture, and animals cannot speak anyway. The point is not to rush into things. Many eager surfers blindly charge into the ocean only to realize once it is too late that conditions are not what they expected, they are in the wrong spot, or there is a much easier way of paddling out. In other words, take your time, watch what is going on, and soak it all in.

Let us first consider the process of getting to the lineup. You want to make it out, and when you eventually do, you want to save enough energy to catch some waves. With any sort of substantial surf, getting from shore to the takeoff spot can be a chore. Longer boards make it easier to catch waves but more difficult to punch through a wave. Therefore, each wave that hits you knocks you that much further from your goal. Take enough waves to the head, and you will feel as if you just went through a laundry cycle.

Watch other surfers paddle out, and you might notice a method to their madness. If they are getting clobbered, do not follow their lead. If they zip out with dry hairdo intact, they are likely on to something. At some spots, typically sand-bottom areas with waves breaking all over, paddling out can be a crapshoot. More often than not there is a deepwater channel, a keyhole through the reef, a rip current, or at least a place where the waves are less consistent, therefore making it easier to paddle out. The extra time spent watching can mean the difference between having your session end before it begins and scooting into the lineup unscathed.

Another item to consider before entering the water is your final destination, or the spot in the lineup where you will catch waves. Watch where and how the waves are breaking and try to decide on a spot to set up camp. Pick your peak, and find some landmark along the beach that lines up with it, preferably something large enough to be seen from the water. Hotels, dunes, lifeguard stands, umbrellas, and beach chairs all make suitable markers. Lining up serves multiple purposes. First, if there is not already a pack of surfers on the peak, a landmark shows you where to sit after paddling back after a ride. Waves tend to break in the same spot due to the bottom contours of the area. Second, and especially important for beginners, currents can pull you one way or the other along the shore without you realizing you're moving. After a session you could return to the beach and have no idea where you left your stuff. A landmark makes it obvious when you are drifting.

Rules of the Road

In a nutshell, etiquette boils down to respect. Give it, and you will usually get it. Since there are no hard and fast rules in surfing, it is up to surfers to have some standards. The responsibility falls on us to civilize the lineup. When we fail, people get hurt. At the very least, ignoring these unwritten laws will earn the perpetrator a one-way ticket to Kookville.

Here are some helpful hints to remember whenever you go surfing:

Don't get greedy – Waves have rolled toward shore since the beginning of time, and they will keep coming as long as the earth is spinning.

However, a finite number of waves will break during your session. Do not try to catch every wave you see. At many spots there exists a clear pecking order of locals who, over time, have established their place in the lineup. As a newcomer, you start at the bottom of the food chain. Some beginners commit a major gaffe by paddling directly into a crowded lineup on a giant board and sitting beyond the pack. Or, some greedy surfers paddle around the person in position to steal an approaching wave. This is known as "snaking." Oh, and girls, no matter how cute, should adhere to the same standards as the boys.

Hold onto your stick – Do not discard your board or release it from your grasp during your session. The only time you should lose contact with your surfboard is during a wipeout. In extremely large surf you may have no choice, but for the most part you should be able to hang on. Abandoning ship leads to injuries when waves slam boards into unsuspecting surfers. Your board is your lifeline. Not only will it keep you above water, your board offers the fastest and easiest transportation back to shore. Learn to duck dive or turtle turn. The more time you spend on your board, the sooner you will learn to control it.

Don't worry, be happy – Some surfers complain about everything. "This place sucks." "There aren't any waves around here." "Look at all those kooks." These whiners wear waterproof chips on their shoulders. They misplace their anger at not being able to surf by screaming at the waves. That's right, like a drunken parent abusing a child after a bad day at work, they take their aggression out on the surf. They slap and yell at the water, even flipping the bird at a poor, unsuspecting wave that failed to make them look like a pro. Just once, I would love to see the mistreated wave rear up and smash one of these kooks into the sand.

You represent all of us – When you pick up a surfboard, you become a representative of surfing. Remember, less than one percent of the population surfs. Therefore, most people do not encounter surfers on a regular basis. Any surfer they see represents surfing. It is a lot of responsibility, I know. So don't be a kook. On the way to the beach, help an old lady cross the street. When walking along the sand, stop to pick up some trash. Say "hello" to the fisherman and wish them good luck. "Wow," they will think, "them surfers ain't so bad."

Kooks are people, too – No one chooses to be a kook. They deserve compassion. When you see someone fumbling through a breach of etiquette, put yourself in his booties for a moment. If he is in over his head, kindly let him know. Kooks can use a helpful nudge in the right direction. If he is doing something stupid, he needs our help. We have all been there.

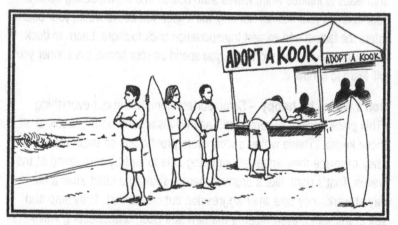

HELPING A KOOK BECOME A BETTER SURFER WILL MAKE YOU A BETTER PERSON.

CHAPTER 4 - GET AN EDUCATION

In This Chapter
Do It Yourself
Private Lessons
School of Surf
Surf Clubs and Organizations
Things I Wish Someone Had Told
    Me When I Started

I have provided you with the fundamentals of surfing over these first few chapters. Unless you possess a photographic memory, you have already forgotten a good portion of it. Unfortunately, I cannot float above your shoulder in a bubble to remind you when you are being a kook. You could try laminating a cheat sheet and taping it to your wrist like a quarterback's playlist, but even then you would have trouble pinpointing your own weaknesses. Doing it on your own is admirable, but there are other options.

The surfing education process can be easy or difficult, fast or slow, cheap or expensive. Where your experience falls on this spectrum can be attributed to what avenue you choose, but it also depends on you. Some people appear hardwired for surfing. They stand up on their first wave and look as casual as if they are walking down the sidewalk. Others, unfortunately, look as if they could not stand on an ocean liner, much less a surfboard. It helps to be limber, strong, athletic, and coordinated. None of these traits, however, are imperative, and each can be developed over time.

How will you go about learning to surf? Let's look at your options.

Do It Yourself

Going at it alone is undoubtedly the slowest method of learning to surf. A solo mission can be lonely and frustrating. There may be times you believe Mark Twain was correct when, after trying

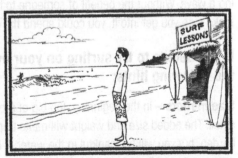

ALONG MOST BEACHES WHERE THERE IS SURFING, THERE ARE PEOPLE WILLING TO TEACH YOU HOW TO SURF.

to surf in Hawaii in 1872 and failing miserably, he insisted, "None but natives ever master the art of surf-bathing thoroughly." What Twain would have found, had he stuck with it, was that anyone can surf. For some people the process takes longer than for others. The reasons for slow improvement might be improper equipment, unpredictable conditions, or any number of individual mistakes.

Nobody taught me how to surf. At age 12, I went out with some friends who had been at it a while and followed their lead. After several sessions, I still could not stand up. Eventually that summer I made it to my feet, but I did not surf during the ensuing winter and had to learn all over again the following spring. No one gave me a beginner board to ride, nor did I receive any pushes into waves or critiques of my faults. Meanwhile, I never asked for or wanted any help. That is just me. I wanted to conquer this challenge on my own, and I did.

The most important things you miss out on by going solo are the use of an appropriate beginner board and a push. That first issue is easily remedied by checking surf shops or rental stands for a proper starter board. Getting pushed into waves, on the other hand, can make all the difference in the world. Often the most difficult part of learning to surf is simply catching a wave. Without the benefit of someone to handpick your wave and make sure you get into it, you could spend the entire session floundering.

If you decide to try surfing on your own, at least consider the following hints:

Size matters – In the beginning, too big of a board is better than too small. The added size and weight will make transporting the beast quite a burden, but you will be thankful in the water. A longer board catches waves more easily and is more stable when you attempt to stand. You can always graduate to a smaller board later.

Location, location, location – The type of lineup and surf conditions for your initial sessions can mean the difference between returning to landlubbing and surfing for life. Try to find a "user-friendly" break when starting out, with gently sloped waves that roll for at least several seconds before reaching shore. And stay away from crowds. You have enough on your plate without a bunch of boards aimed at your head.

Get busy on the sand – Practice several surf-ups on dry land before attempting to ride a wave. Unless you spring out of bed each morning like a fireman, your body is probably not used to popping up like this. Gradually, muscle memory will take over, and you will hardly need to think about what you are doing.

Private Lessons

At most surfing beaches, you can find an experienced local surfer willing to provide instruction in the fundamentals of riding waves. A good surfer does not necessarily make a good teacher. Teaching requires the ability to express ideas clearly, as well as a healthy dose of patience.

A vast amount of information can be passed on during a single lesson, which typically lasts for an hour or two. A talented instructor can demonstrate the proper method of paddling out and standing up, as well as some safety tips, within the first few minutes. Wanting to get in the water in a hurry is understandable, but be patient. Listen to what he has to say. The next step should consist of the student being helped into the lineup and pushed into some waves. At the conclusion of each wave, the rider flips around and paddles to meet the instructor back in the lineup. If paddling out proves too difficult, the instructor will wade in to assist. The instructor watches each ride and offers constructive criticism. Among the benefits of one-on-one instruction, the student gets an opportunity to ride lots of waves, far more than if he had ventured out alone. Some instructors stand on the beach and bark out instructions like a Little League dad. If you feel safer having someone in the water, be sure to ask beforehand.

The best place to begin a search for a qualified instructor is the local surf shop, preferably one that stocks surfboards and not just tourist items. The shop probably has an employee, a team rider, or someone they recommend. The instructor should provide the use of a surfboard with both safety and ease of use in mind. Soft boards offer the safest route and are ideal for a first lesson. If the only thing available is a fiberglass board, make sure there are no jagged areas that could injure the rider in the event of a wipeout. A round nose, rather than a pointed one, means added safety and stability. For a beginner, the board needs to be somewhere between two and four feet longer than the height of the rider.

Cost varies greatly depending upon the area and qualifications of the instructor. A one-hour lesson, surfboard included, usually runs from $30 to as much as $200 in some ritzy areas. At the low end of the scale, the instructor is usually a younger surfer with limited experience. Youth is not necessarily a bad thing in terms of a teacher, as many youngsters provide a wealth of enthusiasm and energy. More experienced instructors tend to charge more for their services and bring with them a proven track record of successful students. Be sure to ask around town before settling on a teacher, and do not hesitate to ask for references.

School of Surf

The number of surf schools has dramatically increased in recent years, making it a common avenue for fledgling surfers. Armies of softboard-dragging newbies magically appear each summer to choke out lineups along every coast of the United States and beyond. During the course of a few fun-filled, action-packed days, students are given a crash course in surfology. Under the right tutelage these students can pick up a few years' worth of education in less than a week. Many summer surf "camps" are geared towards 'tweens and teens, while some schools conduct sessions exclusively for adults, girls, or other groups. For those who live far from any beach, some schools offer overnight camps that include room and meals. Some camps are located in tropical climates and operate on a year-round basis, so your surfing education is not restricted to summertime.

When searching for a surf school, here are some characteristics to look for:

Low student/instructor ratio – There should be at least one instructor for every five students. Any less, and keeping track of everyone becomes difficult.

Instructors aren't paid to surf – Surfing requires complete focus. If an instructor is surfing, he is probably doing his job. I say "probably" because expert instructors sometimes use a surfboard as a tool to help them keep up with their students or for demonstration purposes. Toward the end of camp, it is okay for the instructors to surf with the students. Doing so can be fun for both parties, and it lets the students see that they are learning from real surfers.

Differentiated instruction – Some programs are more like oceanic day care. They might push the kids into a few waves in the beginning, but the rest of the time the students are on their own. A solid program will split students into groups according to skill level and help each surfer progress. Intermediate students should get help with maneuvers.

Instructors are CPR certified – While they will probably not ever have to use CPR on a student, being certified means that instructors take their job seriously.

They can provide references – Previous customers can tell you exactly what each school does well and not so well.

Surf Clubs and Organizations

If the notion of surfing in competition gives you the willies, you are not alone. There are many gatherings of surfers that have nothing to do with contest jerseys or judges. They allow you to meet others who love to surf without worrying about points and trophies. Some are simply social networks, while many congregate for a purpose such as environmental preservation, beach access, or any other cause. Clubs can represent schools, surf shops, local beaches, or much larger entities.

The best-known surfing organization is the Surfrider Foundation, a non-profit group founded in 1984 that has since expanded worldwide. Their stated mission is to protect the planet's oceans, waves, and beaches. They have won massive cases against polluters, blocked projects that threatened to ruin surfing spots and beaches, held thousands of local beach clean-ups, and helped educate children about the importance of preserving our natural environment. As a surfer, you owe it to Mother Nature to assist in her wellbeing. By banding together, surfers have proven they are a force to be reckoned with.

Things I Wish Someone Had Told Me When I Started

In addition to understanding how to surf, there are some other basic points that are helpful to know in the beginning. I was clueless about these things when I started. Eventually you may figure everything out through trial and error, but why not save yourself some trouble and potential embarrassment.

There's a right and a wrong way to wear a wetsuit – The first time I went surfing, I put my wetsuit on backwards. Getting in and out of a wetsuit can be a grueling ordeal, especially on the beach when it is cold outside. I did not think it was very funny, but my friends found my little mix-up hilarious. Try your wetsuit on at home to make sure you know which way is correct. Many diving wetsuits have zippers in front, while most surfing suits have a zipper on the back.

The fins point into the water, not out of it – Having never seen anyone surf, I assumed the side of the board with the fins on it is supposed to face upwards. That way the board would look like a shark traveling through the

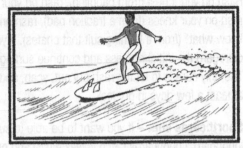

"WHAT DO YOU MEAN THE FINS AREN'T SUPPOSED TO BE FACING UP? BUT, ISN'T THAT HOW SHARKS DO IT?"

water. It made perfect sense to me. Fortunately, I learned of my misunderstanding before actually hitting the water. Otherwise I would have—well, I don't want to think what might have happened.

Wind direction explains where the wind is coming from, not where it's going – The wind greatly affects the surf, so surfers naturally become amateur weathermen, some more quickly than others. A west wind does not blow west. It blows from the west toward the east. This seemingly minor oversight becomes meaningful when your dad drives you several hours to surf based on your weather report. I had this minor point completely backwards for a couple years before figuring it out the hard way.

Water does not provide sun protection – Everybody knows you need sunscreen when you are lying on the beach, but I assumed application before surfing was unnecessary. I would be in the water after all, so I would be covered. Well, on my first surf safari to Florida, I was covered . . . with blisters. Water does not protect skin from the sun at all. Mine had to peel off for me to learn this lesson.

Get used to having a rash – As a surfer, you learn to live with rashes. Rash on your chest (from paddling), rash on your armpits (from a wetsuit), rash on your knees (from a traction pad), rash on your . . . um, your "you know what" (from a bathing suit that chafes). If you are like me, you will disregard the initial redness and continue surfing until you are bleeding. The only cure is to let the rash dry out, scab, and heal on its own, meaning at least a few days in drydock.

Shortboards sink – If you want to be able to surf immediately, ride a longboard. Longboards catch waves easily and provide plenty of stability. Shortboards, on the other hand, are slow at paddling and wobbly when surfing. Sure, shortboards look cool under your arm on the way down the beach, but they are not made for beginners.

CHAPTER 5 - SURFER BEWARE

In This Chapter

Of all the reasons people concoct to avoid learning to surf, the worst is, "It's too dangerous." In reality, horseback riding and cheerleading are far riskier. Among the so-called "extreme" sports, surfing is the old granny of the bunch. It is the oldest and the safest. Big-wave riding is another story, but 99 percent of what we consider surfing fails to live up to the myth of being a treacherous pursuit.

Still, there are many things that can go wrong in the water. Injuries occur, running the entire gamut between a minor crab pinch and the extremely rare fatality. The power and unpredictability of the ocean should never be taken lightly. But if you know what to expect, and keep your cool, you can avoid most potential disasters. In this chapter we will examine scenarios that could turn a great day at the beach into a bummer.

Your Own Worst Enemy

Pick up your surfboard and look in the mirror. You see that wannabe surfer staring back at you? That kook and his board could be the greatest threats to your wellbeing. The danger is not the massive wave, the razor-sharp reef, or the hungry shark. Those things are scary, but you might never encounter them. That pair in the mirror will be with you for every moment of your surfing life. Believe me, they can be dangerous.

The path to safety starts with building a relationship with your surfboard. A board should not be viewed as some weird foreign uncle who smells funny. Your surfboard is your friend. Treat it with respect, and it will bring you great pleasure and possibly save your life. Be mindful of how you carry your board into the ocean, how you accompany it into an oncoming wave, and how you deal with it when all hell breaks loose.

Always carry your board at your side when entering the water. That way, the nose of the board points directly into an approaching shorebreak wave and will penetrate. If you hold the board in front of you, between your body and the wave, you are likely to get knocked over.

While paddling through a wave, it is equally important to keep the board pointed straight out to sea. You are the captain of this ship and must assume responsibility for keeping it afloat. If a wave hits you broadside, you are going to flip. Point toward the horizon, and the chances of emerging on the other side unscathed increase dramatically.

Any time you are riding a wave and find yourself falling or needing to eject, never push your board into your impending path. If you do, your momentum may get you gored by your fins. Instead, try pushing your board off to the side as far out of the way as possible.

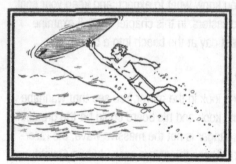

Finally, when you find yourself underwater and separated from your board, *always* let your hands lead the way back to the surface. Cover your head! If by

WHEN UNDER WATER, ALWAYS LEAD WITH YOUR HANDS ON THE WAY UP.

some chance your board is above you, you do not want to head-butt one of your fins.

Crowds

As much harm as you can do to yourself, imagine the wrath of an entire lineup of people just like you. Surfing in crowds, even in small waves, can be downright dodgy. As if learning to surf is not difficult enough, boards are flying around like spears at the Zulu Olympics. It pays to enter the fray with a plan.

I said this earlier, but remember not to get in anyone's way. Paddle around the lineup rather than straight through it. Beware of runaway surfboards, because the sooner you spot one coming your way, the easier it is to avoid it. If you do not see it coming until it is too late, try deflecting the oncoming board with your hand. When that is not feasible, dive for cover or as a last resort use your board as a shield. Better to get a ding in your board than in your body.

Begin at the fringe of the crowd rather than plunging into the middle of it. That way you can assess the situation and gradually ease into the rotation. It may be that there are only a few waves coming through every hour, and joining the starving throng would be futile. Ideally, there are plenty to go around and no one will look at you as yet another vulture scavenging for scraps. When everyone is getting waves, nobody minds sharing.

If you venture out at a spot for the first time, be mindful of your status as an outsider. Many locals do not take kindly to visitors of any sort, especially not greedy ones. Never paddle out and start calling people off waves even if you find yourself in position. You can get a sense of the tension level in the lineup by attempting to strike up a conversation. If the other surfers throw you a stink-eye or ignore you altogether, you may want to mosey along to another peak. There are enough spots where the surfers are friendly that there is no sense in trespassing where you are not wanted.

Laws

The only official rules to surfing are those imposed by local governments in order to protect the rights of swimmers or the wellbeing of surfers. Possible ordinances include complete or partial bans on surfing, a mandatory leash law, or an order to stay a certain number of feet away from a pier, jetty, inlet, or other structure. Occasionally authorities will close a beach due to extremely rough conditions or dirty water. Fines for breaking these laws can cost as much as a few hundred dollars, and ignorance is no excuse. If no signs are posted regarding restrictions on surfing, do not be afraid to ask around before paddling out.

Currents

Awareness about currents prior to entering the water is imperative. For experienced surfers, currents can be used as tools for an easy paddle out or a conveyor belt ride to a better position in the lineup. For beginners, they can prove disastrous.

Longshore currents run parallel to the shoreline. Depending on the daily conditions, these currents can vary from barely noticeable to a river of rushing water. In stormy surf, longshore currents are at their strongest and most dangerous. They can carry a surfer hundreds of yards along the shore in a short time. On days in which the conditions appear relatively tame, these currents can potentially drag surfers into hazardous situations such as close contact with piers or jetties.

The best way to avoid the pitfalls of longshore currents is to be aware of their existence and plan accordingly. Before entering the surf, watch other surfers to see if they are drifting. Walk along the shore against the current before paddling out. That way you will drift back to where you started. Finding a landmark along the beach is important when dealing with longshore currents in order to keep track of your position. Paddling against currents is tiring and sometimes useless. To break free of a longshore current's grip, paddle toward the shore.

Rip currents contrast from longshore currents in that they run out to sea rather than along it. These frequently misunderstood currents are often responsible for drowning swimmers who expend their energy in a futile struggle.

Rip currents are visibly choppier than the surrounding waters and possess an obviously outward flow. They don't run out to sea indefinitely, instead stopping just beyond the outermost line of breakers. To escape from the pull of a rip current, swim or paddle in a direction perpendicular to the shoreline. In other words, paddle across the

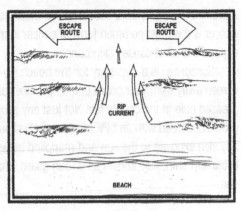

UNDERSTANDING RIP CURRENTS IS A MUST FOR ANY SURFER.

current instead of against it. They are not too wide, perhaps twenty feet across, so getting out isn't difficult.

Remember, you are better off on a surfboard than abandoning ship and attempting to swim to safety. While swimming, you are constantly using energy to stay afloat. On a surfboard, you can rest occasionally without going under. The added elevation also makes it easier to look around and determine to best plan of escape.

Sun Exposure

There's an older surfer in my hometown that noticed an abnormal lesion on his lip a few years ago. His dermatologist decided to remove a chunk of the guy's lip and replace it with a skin graft from another place on his body. Rumor has it that other place turned out to be his butt, earning this fellow the unflattering nickname "Butt Lip." Don't be a Butt Lip. Wear sunscreen. I know several surfers who have developed skin cancer as a result of their time in the sun. The Butt Lip story is scary, but it doesn't represent the worst-case scenario. Too much sun can literally kill you. Skin cancer is the most common form of cancer in the United States, and sun exposure is what causes skin cancer.

Sunscreen is a necessity for the beach. By the way, keep the sunscreen away from your board unless you like your deck as slippery as a greased pole at the county fair. Not just any sunscreen will do. A waterproof sunscreen with an SPF of at least 15 should be applied liberally to any skin exposed to the sun and reapplied between sessions. In addition, a Lycra surf shirt, also known as a rash guard, provides protection from the sun.

Critters

How would you feel if your house were turned into a playground? What if hordes of people descended upon your yard and trampled all over your roses? Would you become territorial if a bunch of dudes danced around your living room while you were trying to watch *American Idol*? The ocean is home to all sorts of creatures that are, for the most part, nice enough to let us frolic in their humble abode.

Sharks are the ocean dwellers with the most potential to make the hair on the back of our necks stand up. They do, after all, eat people. Right? Well, not usually. According to statistics compiled by the International Shark Attack File, one person dies from shark-inflicted wounds in the United States every two years. Considering that gazillions of people play in the ocean (close to 300,000,000 annually), half-a-person each year isn't bad. Sharks kill less frequently than mountain lions, and the shark-induced body count doesn't come close to that of snakes or dogs.

There are surf spots where shark attacks occur with more regularity, mainly in parts of Northern California and Central Florida. For the most part, these encounters seem to be cases of mistaken identity. Once the shark realizes the surfer is not a fish or seal, they tend to continue searching for lunch elsewhere.

Sea urchins are found along coral reefs and can pose a serious threat when stepped on. These small, bulbous critters are covered with sharp spines that can penetrate the flesh and become infected. Urchins won't come looking for you, but it is important to keep an eye on the reef and watch where you step.

Sea lice are particularly nasty little blobs of jellyfish larvae that itch like the dickens. They show up periodically in summer and can ruin a session. They pose no danger but can clear a lineup of surfers faster than a tsunami.

Along the East Coast of the United States, jellyfish are as widespread as tourists in summer. Typically, jellyfish stings constitute just a minor inconvenience. Dolphin and porpoise sightings are common in many surf areas. These harmless animals love to swim in the surf zone and will ride waves on occasion. Other sea critters include skates or stingrays, fish, and crabs. None is particularly menacing. In fact, no sea creature poses as much of a risk to your safety as your own board.

Obstructions

Skateboarders love obstacles; surfers do not. We already have everything we need. Waves are Nature's skateparks, providing pipes, rails, banks, and bowls. Meeting an obstacle in the water is an accidental encounter that usually doesn't end well. Surf spots contain all sorts of objects that need to be avoided.

Piers, jetties, and groins are a few of the man-made structures commonly found in surf zones. Sandbars tend to form alongside these structures, making them magnets for surfers. Here it is helpful to understand the currents, because nobody enjoys being swept into one of these

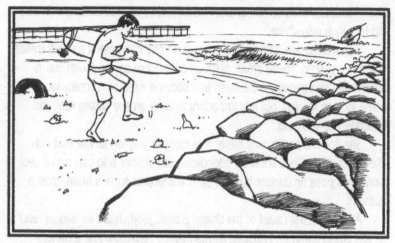

SOMETIMES, JUST GETTING TO THE WATER IS THE HARDEST PART OF SURFING.

immovable objects. Remain cognizant of where you are in relation to surrounding obstacles at all times.

Other obstructions to be wary of in the lineup include coral reefs, rocks, and even shipwrecks. Each can make for great waves as well as serious danger. These hazards are sometimes visible above the surface but can also lurk undetected beneath it. Boils, or circular areas of turbulence, in the face of a wave may indicate the existence of an underwater obstacle. If you are unfamiliar with the lineup, ask around before paddling out.

Thanks to kooks who litter, the beach can be dangerous too. Partially buried broken bottles, usually from alcoholic beverages, can turn the sand into a warzone. Perpetrators are typically individuals, but big companies have also been known to dispose of their waste in the sea. Medical waste, including used syringes, was turning up on the Jersey Shore a while back. This is the exception rather than the rule, but you have to be careful.

Severe Weather

While sane people smartly head for the hills when faced with an approaching tempest, surfers willingly charge into the sea to greet it. This lust for adventure may border on the absurd, but we can't help it. For many surfers, the wilder the conditions, the happier we become. Still, the ocean is a dangerous place when Nature throws a hissy fit.

Swell heights rise rapidly during a storm, putting unsuspecting surfers in situations for which they are not prepared. Furthermore, storms are usually accompanied by strong winds, pelting rain, and lightning. Heavy wind leads to currents, and reduced visibility in a downpour makes mistakes more common. You rarely hear of a surfer lost at sea under sunny, windless conditions. It is during the dark, drifty days when people get into trouble. Unless you are a very strong paddler, stay away from victory-at-sea conditions.

A little rain won't hurt anyone other than the Wicked Witch of the West, but under no circumstances is it safe to go surfing during a thunderstorm. If you suspect the presence of lightning, get out of the water and off the beach as quickly as possible. You are often the highest point in the water or on the sand, making an easy target for lightning. I know a handful of surfers who have been struck and lived to tell the tale, but that is not always the case. Lightning kills. Take cover, and wait for the storm to pass. The waves are usually better on the backside of the storm anyway.

Leaving the Shore and Getting Back

At many spots hitting the surf takes little effort or forethought, but in some cases success is only achieved through patience and observation. Watch how the locals paddle out or in. Do they trudge a half-mile up the beach and hop in to avoid a pounding out front? Do they jump off a particular rock and shoot right into the lineup? Do they turn their boards upside down to protect their fins and tiptoe across the reef until they reach deeper water? It is always fun to watch some bozo sprint across the beach and dive onto his board only to discover he is in ankle deep water, sending him skidding off the front onto almost dry sand.

Consider how you plan to get back to the beach at the end of your session. Again, this could be a non-issue at your standard sand bottom beachbreak. However, at some spots paddling directly to shore is the last thing you want to do. There could be rocks, reef, or some other menacing obstacle standing in the way. Once you come across that barrier, it might be too late. Waves could be pounding you into a bloody pulp atop a slab of fire coral. It is a gruesome thought, so think about it before you paddle out rather than after.

Wipeout

Everybody falls. Not even the best surfers in the world stayed glued atop their boards forever. If you are not falling on your face, or your rear end, or wherever, then you are not trying anything new. You will wipe out. I promise. Once you learn to go with the flow, you might enjoy crashing on occasion. Wiping out is a skill, and the sooner you become proficient at it, the better off you will be. The greatest dangers involve hitting your board, hitting another surfer, hitting the bottom or some other obstruction, or getting held underwater by the force of the wave.

Wipeouts occur for several reasons. You may get rolled by a wave while paddling out, fall when taking off on a wave, slip during a turn, get whacked by the lip, or just plain keel over. Regardless, how you deal with a wipeout should not change.

Your surfboard is the first consideration. When you feel like you are falling and unable to recover, make every effort to avoid landing on your board. Especially hazardous are the fins and nose (on a shortboard).

Likewise, try not to make another surfer a victim by haphazardly turning your board into a missile. By being aware of these threats, your body will make subtle adjustments on the way down to hopefully find a safe landing spot for you and your board.

An understanding of the lineup includes knowing how deep the water is and what lies beneath it. Are you riding atop two feet of water or ten, and is the bottom made of sand or something more sinister? Never dive headfirst unless you are certain there is enough water to slow your descent. Hitting the bottom can lead to injury, including serious spinal cord damage. In shallow water (less than five feet), try to land with your body flat in order to keep from slamming into the bottom. In deeper water, it is okay to dive.

"HEY, KOOK!" **During a wipeout, do not spazz out.** This is easier said than done, but fighting against the wave's energy usually makes things worse. Panicking uses oxygen, and flailing can keep you entangled in the wave as it moves toward shore. By relaxing, you sink deeper and allow the wave to pass. The deeper you are, the less turbulence you will experience. Once the wave's force moves on, you are clear to return to the surface.

In Over Your Head

All surfers eventually find themselves in a situation where they realize, "Whoa, this is scary. I gotta get out of here." When that surfer is you, all you will care about is reaching the shore alive. Your sole mission in life becomes crawling up the beach and smooching the sand. Here are some tips that will help you achieve that goal:

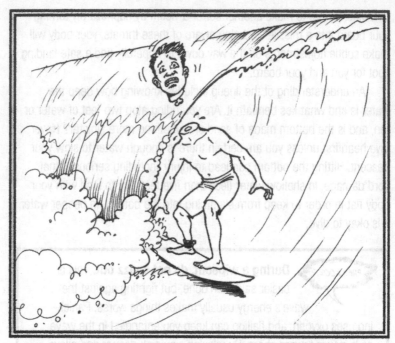

YOU DEFINITELY DON'T WANT TO LOSE YOUR HEAD IN THE WATER.

Use your head – First and foremost, think. Cooler heads will always prevail. Look around and figure out the best route to safety. Only one in every 3.5 million beachgoers drowns, so chances are you will make it.

Stay with your board – Surfboards float, so consider yours as a life raft. Cling to it with all your strength, as it represents your best hope for survival. If you happen to become separated from your board, try flagging down another surfer or a lifeguard by calling out and waving an arm.

Whitewater leads to shore – The obvious instinct in times of distress is to seek calmer water, but that may not be the best option. Rip currents flow through deeper water, which is also where fewer waves break. Therefore, scurrying away from the waves can lead to more trouble. Instead, stay among the waves and have the whitewater push you to shore.

Common Injuries

If you surf long enough, eventually something will go wrong. Here are some common injuries that occur while surfing.

Cuts – The most common accidents are cuts from either a surfboard or the reef. These wounds should be dealt with like any other cuts—wash, pat dry, clean with an antiseptic, and treat with an antibiotic ointment. The ocean helps cuts heal, but they need to dry out in order to mend. Keeping a cut from getting wet while surfing is not easy.

Sunburn – No matter how religiously you apply sunscreen, you will get burned here and there. Aloe plants are great natural healers. Aloe gel works well if you cannot find a plant.

Rash – Wetsuits, boardshorts, and surfboards can cause skin rashes from chafing. Diaper rash ointment works for surfing rashes. Coat the chafed area with Vaseline while surfing to keep it from getting worse. Many surf shops carry a product called Belly Jelly specifically designed for these rashes.

Cramps – Dehydration leads to cramping, which is difficult to treat in the water. Return to the beach and try stretching and massaging the affected area.

Pulled muscle – Twisting and turning atop an unsteady, unpredictable surface can easily result in a pulled muscle. In rare cases, an especially nasty wipeout leads to further damage, including torn ligaments. Obviously, such instances require a visit to the doctor and potential surgery. For minor sprains or strains, refer to the old RICE approach (Rest, Ice, Compression, Elevation).

Surfer's ear – Also known as exostosis, this abnormal bone growth in the ear canal results from prolonged exposure to cold and wind. It is not terribly common, but in some cases the growth completely shuts off the ear canal, leading to hearing loss and possible infection. This ailment requires surgery, whereby a doctor grinds away the additional bone to reopen the canal.

Surfer's myelopathy – Hyperextension of one's back while paddling can cut off the supply of blood to the spine and lead to a rare (roughly one in a million) condition affecting first-time surfers. Victims are left with temporary or occasionally permanent paralysis of the lower extremities. Early warning signs include back pain or stiffness or numbness in the legs or feet.

CHAPTER 6 - SURF SHAPE

In This Chapter

Strength
Flexibility
Balance
Endurance
Mind
Diet

The best exercise you can do for surfing is surfing. There are pro surfers, in fact, who do nothing but surf. No other training whatsoever. These are professional athletes who are in supreme physical condition, and all they do, all they have ever done, is surf. Still, there are several non-surfing activities that can help increase proficiency in the water. They can make surfing safer, easier, and more fun.

Strength

You do not have to be Arnold Schwarzenegger to surf. Excessive musculature hinders flexibility and can make surfing more difficult. Hours spent pumping up in the gym will probably not help you in the water. If you can swim a lap and do a push up, you are powerful enough to get started. Gradually,

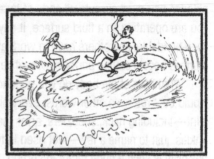

BIG MUSCLES LOOK ATTRACTIVE ON THE BEACH, BUT IN THE WATER THEY CAN GET IN THE WAY OF GOOD SURFING.

time spent surfing will make you stronger by toning muscles in the places you need the extra strength. Avid surfers are, in most cases, extremely fit.

When you are starting out, you will use muscles you never knew you had. For paddling and pushing up, you need some strength in your arms, shoulders, and back. Practicing and mastering the "Surf-Up" (Chapter Two) offers the best preparation. If you have trouble jumping to your feet, start with simple push-ups until you can pop up quickly enough to get your feet underneath you.

To increase strength for paddling, swimming provides the ultimate exercise, an activity free of impact that strengthens not only the muscles but also the cardiovascular system. A basic front crawl is a good place to start, as it mimics the motions of paddling. The pool is fine, but eventually graduating to ocean swimming will help you acclimate to the conditions. It is a good idea to be able to swim for at least ten minutes without stopping. If you can do that, you are ready to take on the waves.

Flexibility

Far more than brute strength, flexibility is imperative to surfing. Considering you must execute all sorts of twists and bends, not to mention that you are operating on a fluid surface, it pays to be flexible. Some people are born bendable, and others have to work at it. Either way, you need it. Suppleness boosts surfing performance while helping to avoid injuries.

What area of the body do you need to stretch for surfing? That answer would be, "Yes"—in other words, everything. Most every muscle and joint—including neck, shoulders, arms, hands, back, hips, legs, knees, and ankles, just to name a few—get used in the act of riding waves. Because flexibility is such a huge factor in surfing, stretching becomes part of the routine. Surfers do not usually stop for anything when the waves are up, yet along the shoreline you often see them pause a few minutes to stretch. (By the way, this offers a prime opportunity to assess the conditions and come up with a plan of action.)

Yoga has become an extremely popular pursuit among surfers for its many cross-training benefits. Beyond merely aiding in flexibility, yoga also increases strength, balance, and focus.

Being loose is of great importance when it comes to wiping out. It is not uncommon to see a surfer's limbs flailing in every direction during a spill. Pulled or strained muscles can be the unfortunate result, especially when your body is stiff. Join a yoga class or at least take a minute to loosen up on the sand prior to paddling out. Your body and your surfing will thank you.

Balance

Standing on a surfboard requires more balance than walking out to the mailbox but considerably less than landing a "backward double salto" on a balance beam. In other words, you are probably okay. If you stand in the right spot on your board, it does most of the work. Still, balance helps. Surfing will improve your balance, but in the meantime, here are some things you can do to jumpstart your sense of equilibrium.

Balance boards are exactly what the name implies: a board that helps develop your balance as well as enhancing core strength. Typically around three feet long and oval or rectangular in shape, they are made of wood and perch atop a rolling cylinder of approximately six inches in diameter. By standing on this unstable contraption, you exercise the same core muscles you use while surfing. They run around $100, or you can try to build it yourself for a fraction of the cost. Balance balls provide a similar workout.

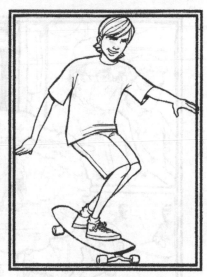

JUST AS WITH SURFING, LONGBOARD SKATING REQUIRES PUMPING TO GENERATE SPEED.

Skateboarding is an excellent way to practice surfing movements and have fun doing it. Longboard skateboards, meant for carving down hills and along streets, are close in nature to surfing. By gyrating your hips and rapidly turning the board back and forth, you can generate speed as you would on a wave.

Endurance

Some days a half-hour session is all you want or can afford, but on those special days when the surf says, "All day," you don't want your body responding, "No way." Believe me, it might be flat today, but the doldrums do not last forever. Meanwhile, take advantage of this time to raise your endurance level. If you cannot go surfing or at least take a paddle, find some other physical activity in which to partake. Go swimming. Take a stand-up paddle. Ride your bike. Run along the beach. Hop on your

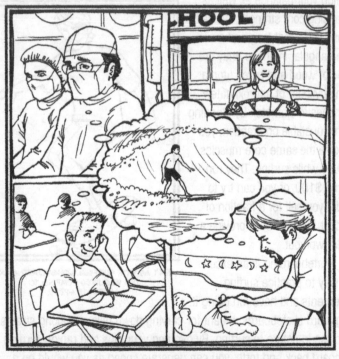

THE MIND REALLY IS A TERRIBLE THING TO WASTE. IF YOU ARE UNABLE TO GET IN THE WATER, TRY THE NEXT BEST THING – MIND SURFING.

skateboard and carve up the streets. Put on a speedo and go rollerblading along the boardwalk. I am kidding about that last one, but please do something.

Mind

Surfing is good for the mind, but how do you get your mind ready for surfing? That is easy—go mind surfing. Laugh all you want, but I believe this can make you a better surfer or at least help you maintain your skills while unable to get in the water. Mind surfing can be done while sitting on the beach staring at empty waves as well as anywhere else, be it the office, or the classroom, or even while enjoying dinner at a Mexican restaurant (the curled up corners of tortilla chips bear a striking resemblance to waves).

Simply envision yourself riding a wave. You can do anything you want on that wave, even things that have never been done. If you are not at the beach, make a wave by curling over the corner of a memo from your boss, or doodling one in the margin of your algebra notebook. Go ahead, surf it however you like—power carves, big airs, deep tube rides.

The other aspect of being mentally prepared for surfing involves your comfort level in the ocean. If you have never been in the ocean, never been so far out you could barely see land, or never been bashed around in the breakers, you might feel a bit apprehensive. This nervousness will make learning to surf exceedingly difficult. Fortunately there is a cure. It is called, "Get out there." The only way to become more comfortable in the ocean is to experience it, so go ahead. Dive in.

Diet

Not to worry, I am not going to forbid you from eating anything but seaweed smoothies and trail mix. Certainly your diet has an affect on your execution in the water as it does with any other physical pursuit. Putting crap in an engine results in crappy performance, and the same goes for your body. However, other than a couple obvious no-nos, follow whatever diet you wish. Just be sure not to paddle out right after Thanksgiving dinner, but not because, as your parents warned you, you will cramp up and drown if you go in the water within an hour of eating. Avoid a big meal before surfing because your stomach will hurt, your reflexes will be dulled, and you will likely burp up whatever you ate. Gross! A light pre-surf snack is wonderful, but try not to overdo it. Unfortunately there is no food that will keep you from being a kook, and there is no food that will make you a superstar. However, if you really want to be able to surf till you are 100, or at least for a few hours at a stretch, the following tips are helpful.

Drink lots of water – Staying hydrated is critical even when you are completely surrounded by water, so try to drink lots of it on land. And if you can help it, try not to drink too much seawater when surfing.

Limit sugar – Snack on fruits and veggies rather than candy bars and sodas. The sugar rush wears off rather quickly and will leave you floundering for energy. Perhaps keep an energy bar or two on the beach so you can paddle in and gas up if you are feeling drained.

Eat less – Gorging after a long surf session is understandable, but try limiting your food intake the rest of the time. Staying trim combined with staying active equals a long, healthy life. And plenty of long, healthy surf sessions.

CHAPTER 7 - MOMMY, WHERE DO WAVES COME FROM?

In This Chapter

CHAPTER 7 – MOMMY WHERE DO WAVES COME FROM?

In This Chapter

What Are Waves?

Anatomy of a Wave

Groundswell vs. Windswell

Surface Conditions

Tides

Sets

Swell Direction

Without waves, there is no surfing. We revert back to being Regular Joes, relegated to a lifetime of kook-dom. Even with waves all around us, it is easy to take these natural beauties for granted. We tend to treat them like a longtime spouse, forever grumbling about their shortcomings and never stopping to show our appreciation for their tireless work and dedication. At least spouses get an anniversary card once a year. Waves get nothing, and they deserve better. To show my thanks, I am devoting not just a chapter to waves, but an entire section.

In this chapter, we will examine the nuts and bolts of waves, including what they are, where they come from, and what makes them tick.

What Are Waves?

Let's not get too technical here. For the sake of simplicity, imagine yourself at a football game, and picture a stadium wave. Some fan decides, "Hey, let's do the wave," and jumps out of his seat with arms stretched to the heavens. The more forceful and vocal the guy is, the more likely the stadium wave will be born. The surge of rising bodies then propagates around the arena, yet the fans do not run laps around the place or move other than to stand up and sit back down. Around the stadium this wave goes, a powerful, flowing swell of citizenry. An ocean wave operates in much the same way. The instigator for wave action is the wind. As it blows, the wind creates wave energy at the ocean surface. And just like the stadium wave, the ocean wave does not literally move across the ocean. Only the energy travels. The individual water molecules rise and fall, afterwards returning to roughly their previous position.

By definition, a wave is "one of a series of ridges that moves across the surface of a liquid." In the ocean, some of these ridges are small, and some are big. Some are messy, and some are smooth. Some are bunched up like passengers on a Bangkok bus, and some spread out like neighbors in the Australian Outback.

A combination of several factors, all in regards to wind, determines the size of a wave. Wind strength, the distance over which it blows (known as "fetch"), and the length of time it blows all play a part. Direction, of course, is also of vital importance, as waves form in the direction the wind is blowing. Any increase in the wind's strength, distance, or time will create bigger waves. The largest waves, therefore, are generated by massive storms churning over the open ocean. One additional factor pertaining to wave size is water depth. Deeper water provides a greater medium from which to form a massive wave.

In characterizing waves, weather reporters often refer to the height, period, and direction from which the waves emanate. Wave height indicates the distance from peak to trough. Wave period indicates a time interval between the arrivals of two consecutive crests measured from a stationary point. For example, you may hear that the waves are six feet (height) at ten seconds (period) out of the west (direction). We will dive into greater detail with these characteristics, and why they matter, later on.

What surfers regard as waves, those curling mounds we ride near the shore, are actually called "breakers," but only by kooks and people in lab coats who have earned the title of "doctor" but will never examine a single patient. The part of the wave we ride represents the last death throes of a swell's long journey, the abrupt final stage of its life. Swells will continue their trek across the ocean, however long that may be, until meeting shallow water. Here, the ocean floor "grabs" the swell, slowing it down as it nears the shore. By slowing, the top part of the wave overtakes the bottom, resulting in a "breaker." But remember, we just call them waves.

Anatomy of a Wave

Swell – wave that has yet to reach shallow enough water in which to break; an unbroken wave.

Peak – crest; highest and steepest point of a wave; first portion of a wave to break as it approaches the shore.

Shoulder – sloped outer edge of a wave, similar to the shoulder along a road.

Face – steep part of wave that remains unbroken; wall.

Lip – pitching upper section of a breaking wave; top of a wave as it cascades downward; also known as the curl.

Bottom – trough; lowest point of a wave.

Section – segment of wave that breaks all at once.

Whitewater – broken portion of a wave that continues rolling toward shore.

Flats – area in front of the trough that has yet to be affected by the wave.

Back – rear side of a wave.

Tube – hollow section within a breaking wave; also known as the barrel; most coveted portion of the wave.

Foamball – somewhat spherical mound of whitewater found at the deepest point inside a tube.

Pocket – steep portion of the wave directly adjacent to the lip or curl; ideal location for riding.

Groundswell vs. Windswell

This sounds like a smackdown cage match between former tag-team wrestling mates turned mortal enemies formerly known as "The Swell Guys." Unfortunately, it is not. But if it were a contest, it would be a huge mismatch. Every surfer knows that groundswell would squash poor little windswell.

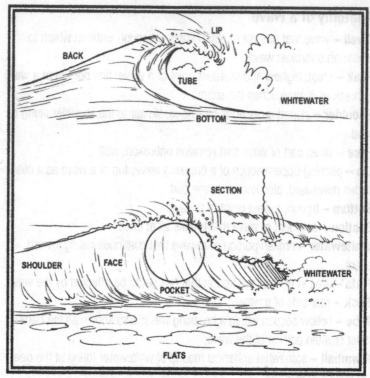

Since swell travels across water and dies abruptly when it reaches any landmass, the term groundswell has nothing to do with the ground. Groundswells originate from storms far out at sea. Because of their gradual development over deep water, these swells form long wave periods and last for anywhere from days to sometimes weeks. They have the potential to produce larger surf that is organized into long lines from its extensive travels across the ocean. The direction of the earth's rotation also plays a role in determining the sort of surf an area receives. Storm systems generally move from west to east around the planet. Therefore, the west coasts of landmasses, as well as islands surrounded by thousands of miles of open-ocean, tend to see more groundswells.

Windswells are waves generated by local winds. By local winds, I mean winds than can be felt along the shore. Windswells are typically short period swells (where waves bunch up one behind another) that quickly fade once the weather system passes.

In smaller bodies of water—such as the Great Lakes, Mediterranean Sea, or Gulf of Mexico—the coastlines receive short period windswell or nothing at all. There is simply not enough of a runway for a groundswell to get moving. Along America's East Coast, windswells constitute the majority of the surf. On occasion this region also receives groundswell, such as with a hurricane that stays far out at sea.

The key differences between groundswells and windswells are the speed and power of the waves they generate. Groundswell waves move faster and arrive at surf spots having built up more power than windswells. Furthermore, the longer periods associated with groundswells create more organized waves. Windswells can be fun, but they lack the magnitude and staying power of groundswells.

Surface Conditions

Wind not only creates waves, it wields the ability to make or break an otherwise promising swell. Local wind conditions make the final determination as to whether the surf is perfect or pitiful. Subtle variations in direction can transform dream scenarios into full-on nightmares. Think of a swell like a car coming through an assembly line. You can equip the vehicle with every feature in the world, but if you leave off the body, you are looking at an ugly heap of metal that no one wants to drive. A swell without an offshore wind is like a car without its body. It has speed, power, and drivability (it gets you where you are going), but it looks like crap and you do not want to ride in it.

Of the 360 degrees from which winds can blow, three-quarters of them create less than ideal conditions. That leaves little room for error. Wind blowing with any velocity from the sides or back of waves wreaks instant havoc on the state of the surf. Sideshore winds cause chops in the wave face and jumpstart a longshore current. Onshore winds, those blowing from the sea toward the shore, do not necessarily ruin the wave face, but they whip the lineup into a disorganized mess that is difficult to ride. Extremely heavy onshore winds produce conditions reminiscent of those found in a washing machine, a dangerous situation known as victory-at-sea.

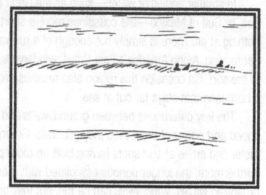

Onshore winds are not all bad. They possess at least one redeeming quality: They make waves. At beaches that do not receive groundswell, the only way to get waves is for the wind to blow hard onshore. The harder it blows, the bigger the waves. Surfers from

GLASSY (ABOVE) VERSUS CHOPPY (BELOW) CONDITIONS. GLASSY WAVES ARE MORE INVITING, BUT SURFING IN ALL CONDITIONS MAKES FOR A WELL-ROUNDED WATERMAN.

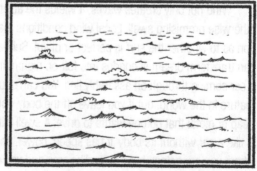

these locales do not mind choppy waves, because without them they would have no waves at all.

Other than simply praying for waves, the one atmospheric circumstance surfers desire is an offshore wind. In order to create the optimum conditions at any particular spot, winds must blow from the land straight out to sea. Offshore winds groom the surface of waves into smooth, slick racetracks that are easy to ride. The overwhelming majority of photos and surf videos are shot under these pristine conditions, often referred to as "clean" or "glassy." Every other day, the wind ranges anywhere from just a bit off to completely whacked

Tides

Tides are critical when it comes to coastal navigation, and these ever-changing oddities are often just as important to surfers. Stemming from the gravitational pull of the moon, the ocean's depth rises and falls twice each day. At some spots, the difference between high and low tide is barely discernable, but waves generally change along with the tide.

An incoming or rising tide usually improves surf conditions. The surge of water adds force to a swell, creating a period of more consistent waves. Once the tide nears its highest point, however, the lineup can become too deep, and waves will break less frequently or cease altogether.

During a dropping tide, a swell becomes smaller and less consistent. On the other hand, some spots only begin breaking when the tide drops. Every lineup has its own nuances based on tides, and the local surfers know exactly when the surf will turn on or off. Watches designed specifically for surfing come with a tide feature, and local tide information can also be found daily in most newspapers or online. Pay attention to the tides, and they will become your friend rather than your enemy.

Sets

A wave is a wave is a wave, right? Wrong. At most any surf break, there are some surfers who sit further out than the rest of the pack. These fellows are either kooks afraid of getting rolled by a breaking wave, or they are the most experienced and skilled surfers in the lineup. The kooks sit way out there because they feel safer in flat water than in an area with consistent wave action. The other surfers—those in the know—sit out there because they are waiting for a "set."

Swells produce waves of varying heights and periods. According to Steve Lyons of the Weather Channel, "As waves move away from the wind source as swell, they sort into more consistent groups of periods." In other words, the longer period waves congregate with other longer period waves, and the short period waves hang out with short period waves, just like cliques of jocks and geeks in high school. As a swell reaches the lineup, it contains a vast range of wave heights. However, the largest waves usually arrive in groups of a couple to a half-dozen or more. These groups are known as sets and tend to break farther out than the average waves. Their arrival is generally consistent and can measure anywhere from every five minutes to once an hour.

Wave knowledge and proper positioning repeatedly put the informed surfer on the best waves, while the ignorant surfer simply cannot figure out how that guy is so darned lucky. The kook keeps getting "caught inside" by the sets and spends his entire session either paddling aimlessly or tumbling underwater. Occasionally, a set of waves comes through that catches even the knowledgeable surfers by surprise. Known as a "clean-up set," this group of exceptionally large waves breaks farther outside than the typical sets and sweeps the lineup clear of surfers. It usually goes unridden.

Swell Direction

Like any veteran surfer, I cannot tell you the number of times my elaborate plans to catch great waves have been thwarted. When I think about all the hours wasted—the preparation and the driving and the moping around kicking the sand—it pains me. What is worse is that I could have avoided most of these heartbreaks just by knowing a little bit about swell direction. Surf science is, after all, not rocket science.

Wind, as you know, creates swell. Whatever direction the wind is coming from dictates the direction, or angle, of the swell. Every surf spot behaves a certain way depending on the swell direction. Each place has what is called a "swell window," a certain section of the compass from which waves are cleared for arrival. If your spot's window is from the north or east, swells from the south or west may not even cause a ripple no matter how powerful they are. The window could be a massive picture window, as with Cape Hatteras sticking way out into the ocean, or it may be a tiny porthole. It all depends on what land, if any, lies off the coast waiting to block potential swell.

If you do not know the ideal swell direction for your beach, ask around or do some research online. The information is not difficult to find. Or, you can be like me and wait until you've been surfing for decades before figuring it out. I managed to "luck" into plenty of great swells through the years, but with a little homework I could have scored at a much higher rate.

PART II: WAVES

CHAPTER 8 – NO TWO WAVES ARE THE SAME

In This Chapter

Right or Left

Beach Break

Point Break

Reef Break

Bunny Slopes or Black Diamonds

Artificial Waves

Weird Waves

My father completely supported my surfing, but he used to give me the hardest time when I asked him to drive the extra five minutes to drop me off at the far end of the beach near the jetty. He refused to believe that the waves there were any different than they were thirty blocks away, where it was far easier to drop me off. It was, after all, the same ocean, the same swell, and the same beach. By spending his formative years shooting pool and looking for fights, he did not get much time in the water. As a result, he failed to understand that the ocean bottom determines how a wave breaks, and the bottom can be vastly different at two locations along the same stretch of beach. Heck, I didn't understand it either. All I knew was that the waves were better next to the jetty, so that was where I had to surf.

Since the ocean bottom—be it sand, reef, or just a bunch of rocks—is what tells a swell how and when to break, it is an area we should know intimately. Everyone gets a free tour of the bottom during a wipeout, but that is not what I am talking about. On a flat day, grab a mask and snorkel and go exploring around the lineup. You will be amazed at what is under there.

In the meantime, we will examine various types of waves and see how and why they differ. Afterwards, you will be able to stride confidently up to the beach and know what you are looking at. Then, you can call my dad and let him know I was right.

Right or Left

There are two ways to eat a banana. You can methodically peel away the skin, leaving the edible inside portion unscathed and ready to be devoured. Or, you can stomp on the banana, spewing its innards all at once. Most people, even some gorillas, choose the former. The same applies to waves. Waves that break abruptly from end to end are not desirable for surfing. They offer a short ride often with time for nothing more than dropping in before the entire wall collapses. These squished bananas of the wave world are called "closeouts." Their opposite is a wave that breaks at its peak and then gradually tapers down the line, providing an open face for riding.

A wave that peels, even for a few brief seconds, is ripe for surfing. These waves are classified as either "lefts" or "rights" depending upon which direction they peel. The determination is made not from the perspective of the beach looking out at the sea, but from the water as if paddling for the wave. This distinction dictates what direction a surfer will ride. When more than one surfer is paddling for a wave, the question of "right or left" is essential.

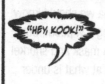

Learn your rights from your lefts. Misreading the direction a wave is breaking can lead to a breach of etiquette, or worse, a collision. Figuring out the best way to go is not difficult. Aim away from the whitewater toward the open face.

Beach Break

The most common surfing lineup is a beach break. At these spots, waves break over a sandbar. Most lineups along the East and Gulf Coasts, along with many West Coast venues, are examples of beach breaks. They generally require less swell and thus break with more consistency than other setups. Often these lineups are ideal for beginners, as they offer mellow waves and a relatively soft landing pad in the event of a wipeout. However, some beach breaks are quite the opposite. Places like Cape Hatteras,

North Carolina; Hossegor, France; and Puerto Escondido, Mexico, are all notoriously powerful and fast-moving beach breaks.

Since sand is continually shifting around the ocean floor in response to waves and currents, beach breaks are known to change periodically. A great lineup can completely disappear overnight due to a powerful storm, and another sandbar may pop up somewhere else along the shore. Jetties, piers, and groins tend to attract sand and maintain it with more efficiency than random stretches of beach, but even these spots are subject to the whims of change.

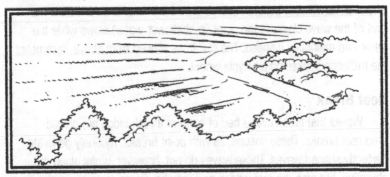

RADIATING OUT LIKE THE SPOKES OF A WHEEL, POINTBREAK WAVES PEEL ALONG FOR OUR SURFING PLEASURE.

Point Break

The regrettable '90s movie of the same name aside, point breaks provide ideal waves for surfing. Typically formed by a rocky outcrop or a curved shoreline such as a bay, point breaks are characterized by long, peeling waves. Whereas beach break rides are often over quickly, point waves allow surfers to stretch their legs and repertoires. The seabed beneath a point break is made up of rocks, and, in some instances, sand. They are common along the California coast, around New England, and across Central

America. Some of the more famous point breaks include Malibu and Trestles in Southern California, Bells Beach and the Gold Coast of Australia, and South Africa's famed Jeffreys Bay. These locations provided the ultimate arenas for surfers through the second half of the twentieth century until being usurped, at least among elite surfers, by ever more challenging outer reefs and mutant slabs around the turn of the millennium. For the majority of surfers, point breaks remain the gold standard.

Swells travel in parallel lines in their journey across the ocean, but upon reaching a point of land or rock, they will bend around it. This phenomenon occurs because waves slow down in shallower water. The part of the wave closer to the point (in shallower water) slows while the other end maintains it speed. The result, as viewed from above, resembles the radiating spokes on a bicycle wheel.

Reef Break

Waves that break over a bed of coral or a rock ledge are considered reef breaks. These lineups, as with point breaks, routinely generate perfectly shaped waves. These waves do not, however, break along the shoreline, but atop the reef wherever it may be. Some reefs are in close proximity to the shore, while others are far out at sea. Mostly located in tropical locations such as Hawaii and Indonesia, reefs create the majority of the pristine yet deadly waves found in surf magazines and movies. Classic examples include Pipeline and Jaws in Hawaii, and Tahiti's infamous Teahupoo. Reef breaks are formed over thousands, sometimes millions, of years and seldom change. Alongside the reef there is usually a deep channel or reef pass that allows for an easy paddle out.

Reef breaks are seldom geared toward novices, as these spots tend to be shallow and carry serious consequences. Waikiki's lineups represent one of the rare exceptions to this rule, boasting several gently breaking "bunny slopes" that are havens for beginners. Simply knowing you are surfing atop a reef can be a harrowing experience. In addition to sometimes being razor sharp, many reefs contain holes or caves that can potentially trap a surfer underwater during a wipeout. It pays to be extra careful when figuring the ins and outs of these dangerous spots. Over time, any competent surfer can learn to surf comfortably and even thrive in these lineups once the initial worry wears off.

Bunny Slopes or Black Diamonds

A novice surfer and an expert wave usually spell disaster. Fortunately, there are plenty of user-friendly waves out there for honing your skills. Trademarks of beginner waves include an easy, sloped takeoff; a slow, peeling manner; a mellow crowd; and a non-threatening seafloor. The majority of surf spots on earth fit these criteria, so you should not have a problem finding your launching pad. The speed at which you graduate to more challenging venues depends on you, but start out slow.

There is no shortage of expert waves on the planet to keep even the bravest of surfers from ever growing bored with the pursuit. As you become more proficient at riding waves, you will seek out more demanding lineups. Bigger waves present an obvious challenge to the fledgling rider, yet size is not the only quality that expert surfers look for in a wave. Basically, highly skilled riders like it steep and deep. The steeper the wave, the more challenging the ride becomes, providing added speed and consequences. By deep, I mean that the ultimate wave does not fold like a cheap suit. It pitches with intense force, creating a hollow void inside the wave. This hollow section is what surfers crave. It is the tube, the Holy Grail of surfing. I will take a hollow five-foot wave over a ten-foot "folder" any day.

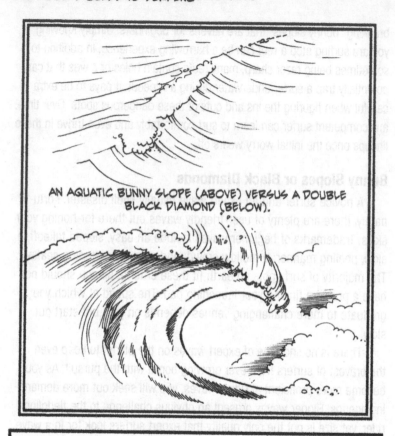

AN AQUATIC BUNNY SLOPE (ABOVE) VERSUS A DOUBLE BLACK DIAMOND (BELOW).

"HEY, KOOK!"

Stick with your kind. If you are learning to surf, look for beginner waves. In more difficult conditions, the lineup will be filled with more advanced surfers. When the waves get heavy, there is less room for error and less tolerance for kooks.

Artificial Waves

For decades, man has tried to recreate ocean waves in pools. To non-surfers who bob around these wave tanks at waterparks across the globe, the enterprise has been a huge success. "Just like the ocean, but without the sand," they blather. But these landlubbers are dead wrong. Surfers know the difference between a man-made wave and a real one. And so far, the two remain leagues apart.

Artificial wave technology has been around since the 1940s, when Palisades Amusement Park in New Jersey used a waterfall at one end of a pool to generate waves. Arizona's "Big Surf" followed in 1969 and was the first to allow surfing. "Big," unfortunately, was a relative term. To a gnome, the surf was overhead. To everyone else, it was waist-high dribble. Since then, heaps of inventive ideas have temporarily captured our imagination in the ongoing quest for the ultimate man-made wave.

Despite pouring millions of dollars into these pools in hopes of pulling millions more out, no one has yet constructed a commercially viable artificial wave. Some have come close, most notably Japan's now defunct Ocean Dome and Disney's Typhoon Lagoon in Orlando. Each has hosted the world's best surfers in competitions before wildly enthusiastic crowds, but history ranks them as novelties rather than legitimate events.

The latest incarnation of artificial waves is the FlowRider, a perpetual "standing" wave generated by shooting water up an inclined plane. One version of the machine creates a wave that looks surfable, but the extremely shallow bottom precludes the use of fins. Therefore, the ride and the equipment are more akin to skimboarding than to surfing.

While far from perfect, the wavelets currently peeling across wavepools make ideal fodder for beginners. Some parks offer surf lessons in these controlled environments, providing a tame introduction to surfing.

Wavepools offer an out-of-the-ordinary surfing experience than can be a fun diversion when the ocean is flat. The day that surfers can drop into the wavepark on the way home from work as easily as hitting the gym, however, remains a pipe dream.

Weird Waves

According to Hawaiian legend, a man named Na Holaua surfed a tsunami during the 1860s. Supposedly, the initial wave swept him from his wooden house and sucked him out to sea, but not before he could rip a plank of wood off the side of his house. As the next massive wave bore down on him, he allegedly turned and stroked into it atop the plank. He then stood and rode the second wave of the tsunami back to shore. Holaua calmly nailed the board back to his house and returned to tending his vegetable garden or whatever else he was doing.

Okay, so I added that last part, but the entire story is far-fetched even from an extreme sports perspective. Tsunamis are typically massive walls of whitewater and thus cannot be ridden. Due to their speed and lack of wave face, they would swamp any potential rider. The thought of riding one of these freaks of nature hardly holds water. There are, however, a few unorthodox types of waves that are in fact ridden.

The need to ride waves has led to the strange phenomenon of river surfing. Taking place in a handful of outposts around the world, this pursuit has grown beyond mere novelty. The waves are technically tidal bores, or the leading edge of the incoming tide. In certain areas—most notably England's River Severn and the Amazon in Brazil—this wall of water forms a decent wave. Given the right conditions, including an especially low tide and a narrowing river bed, these peelers roll for incredible distances. The longest recorded ride in surfing history, in fact, took place in 2003 on a section of the Amazon called the Rio Guajara. Brazilian surfer Picuruta

Salazar rode for 37 minutes straight.

Some rivers, most notably the Snake River running through the American West, generate rideable stationary waves. At certain spots along the river, the flow of water hits upon an outcrop of rock to form a standing wave. These waves can theoretically be ridden forever. However, your legs will cramp up within the first few minutes of constant riding and you will need to kick out for some rest.

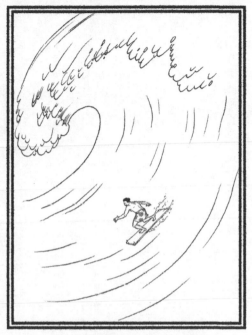

TSUNAMI SURFING ISN'T HAPPENING, NOT ON A SURFBOARD OR A PLANK OF WOOD.

Another interesting place that surfers have found waves is behind tankers, most notably in Texas's Galveston Bay. Here, groups will load their boats with boards and stalk oil tankers around the bay. When they spot a wake worthy of riding, they dive in and catch it. These waves, like river bores, are known to go on for miles.

PART II: WAVES

CHAPTER 9 - WAVES NEAR AND FAR

In This Chapter

PART II: WAVES

CHAPTER 9 – WAVES NEAR AND FAR

In This Chapter
Surf Forecasting
Surf Report
Judging Wave Height
Surf Travel

"How were the waves?"
"How are the waves?"
"How are the waves gonna be tomorrow?"

Ask these questions to a group of surfers, and you may get a different answer from each person. You might think that the first two at least are cut and dry, but in reality all are open to interpretation. The time someone surfs, where he surfs, how many waves he catches, and how he rides them each play a part in how he views the conditions. Despite all the confusion, surfers still ask the questions of one another regularly. And they will continue to ask them as long as they surf. Hopefully, with a little explanation, we can all get on the same page.

Surf Forecasting

Nothing had a bigger impact on surfing around the new millennium than the rise in access to surf forecasting brought about by the Internet. Nowadays, thanks to this technology, no one has an excuse for missing a swell. While far from an exact science, surf forecasts interpret complicated government buoy readings and computer swell models to paint a pretty clear picture of the near future. And it is all a mouse click away.

Much of the information used in surf forecasting comes from NOAA, the National Oceanic and Atmospheric Administration. Established in 1970, this US Department of Commerce agency is tasked with warning us about dangerous weather, charting the seas and skies, and guiding the understanding and protection of the environment. All are important chores, but what we really care about are their projections in regard to the seas. WAM charts (Wave Amplitude Models) offer the key ingredients of wave height and direction. These color-coded maps forecast up to 120 hours (five days) into the future, and they are animated into colorful little cartoons.

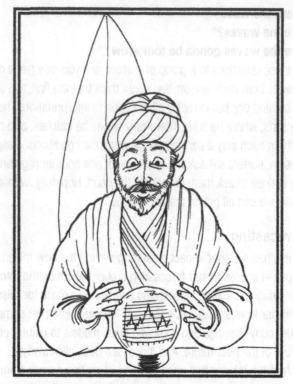

AS SURF FORECASTING HAS BECOME A MORE ACCURATE
SCIENCE, SURFERS HAVE LEARNED TO PLAN THEIR SCHEDULES
AROUND THE PREDICTIONS OF WAVE PROPHETS.

Learning to find and read the WAM charts can make you a surf
forecaster in your own right, but there are plenty of professionals out
there who do the work for you. Among them, Surfline is the granddaddy
of forecasting. Started by California surfer Sean Collins in 1984, Surfline
revolutionized the pursuit of riding waves by telling us when, where, and
how big those waves would be. Sometimes detested for making things too

easy and leading to lineup congestion, few surfers can honestly say they have completely neglected these services. Collins unfortunately passed away in 2011, but surf forecasting, however accurate, is here to stay.

Surf Reports

As long as there have been surf shops (beginning in the 1950s), there have been surf reports. These stores were created to sell surfboards, but their proximity to the ocean bombarded them with the question, "How's the surf?" Shop owners rejoiced in the 1970s when telephone answering machines hit the mainstream, allowing them to record a surf report first thing in the morning. The rest of the day could be spent trying to move product instead of fielding phone calls from inquisitive inlanders. Throughout the ensuing decades, shop reports remained the go-to for surf checks. Nowadays, like everything else, surf reports are almost exclusively online.

Live streaming surf cameras, for obvious reasons, have all but replaced the old recorded surf reports of yore. There are cameras aimed at most major surf spots, transmitting instant images to the World Wide Web. No longer do we have to place our faith in the guy at the surf shop. He could be lying, either telling us that the waves are flat since he is bitter about being stuck in the store all day, or that it is great so we stop in and buy a new board.

A quick glance at the webcam, and we now know exactly how the waves are and how many people are surfing. The result of these continuously updated streaming surf reports is that fewer waves go unridden. From your cubicle or library, you are able to see precisely when the swell hits, but then again, so can everyone else.

Judging Wave Height

There are two ways of stating the size of the surf at any given time—comparing the height of the wave to a human ("It's head-high out there") or estimating the height in feet ("It's six feet out there"). The former is fairly obvious, except of course it depends upon the height of the human. Basically, size up the person who is conveying the information and use his height as a guide. The latter method, assigning a number to the size of the surf, is a dangerous undertaking. Everybody seems to use a different scale, so waves that are six feet to one person might be considered three feet by another surfer or eight feet by the next.

The worst perpetrators of misjudgment and confusion are the very people who delivered modern surfing to the rest of the world: the Hawaiians. Since they were so generous in sharing their favorite pastime, perhaps we should cut them some slack. They are anything but generous when it comes to judging wave height, typically cutting the actual height in half. A wave that measures ten feet high on the face rates as a mere five-footer using the modest Hawaiian scale. Hawaiians derive their number from a rough measurement of the back of the wave, a nonsensical approach if ever there was one. After all, surfers ride the front of the wave, even in Hawaii. The back of the wave is essentially meaningless.

Surfers along the East Coast, possibly because they are so thankful to get waves and careful not to belittle the meager gifts they receive, tend to rate waves for their actual height on the face. A six-foot wave is a six-foot wave. Californians, meanwhile, exercise a scale that is somewhere between that of the East Coast and Hawaii. To further muddy the waters, in Europe and Australia, you often hear waves judged in meters. Without a table for converting meters to feet, who knows what is meant by a 1.5-meter wave? I would explain it to you, but I was absent that day.

Since riding a wave requires complete focus, it is easiest to measure a wave when watching another surfer riding it. Still, sizing up waves is an inexact science. The best way to portray the surf accurately may be to use your hand and say, "It was about yea big."

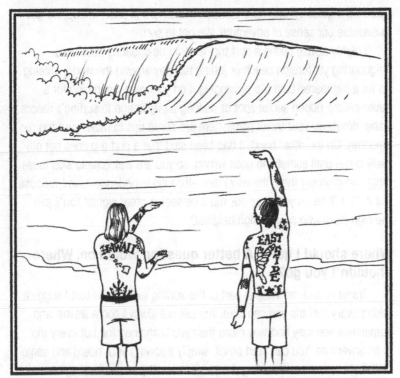

EVERYONE HAS HIS OWN SCALE WHEN IT COMES TO JUDGING WAVES.

Surf Travel

Most people look at a globe and dream of traveling to exotic, faraway places, but as surfers, we experience an especially heightened sense of wanderlust. Waves are breaking right now all over the world, and we wish we could ride all of them. Along with the obvious benefits of foreign travel—learning about foreign cultures, sharing camaraderie with our travel partners and others we meet along the way, and accruing lifelong memories—we as surfers get so much more. While other tourists are following a guide on and off a tour bus like a herd of pasty sheep, we get to exercise our sense of adventure. We get to surf.

I highly advise taking a surf trip. It could be shooting down to a neighboring yet foreign beach or jetting halfway around the world, anteing up for a pampered boat trip or winging it on your own, searching for a never-before-ridden secret spot or making a pilgrimage to surfing's mecca, Oahu. Whatever your travel plans, here are some tips to make your trip run smoothly. On the other hand, it has been said that a surf trip does not officially begin until something goes wrong, so you are welcome to skip these hints and discover them the way I did—through experience. Like Dr. Seuss put it, "You'll be on your way up! You'll be seeing great sights! You'll join the high fliers who soar to high heights!"

Where should I go? – A better question would be, Where shouldn't you go?

Travel is such an integral part of the surfing experience that I suggest taking every surf trip you can take. You will not always score waves, and sometimes you may find way more than you bargained for, but every trip is an adventure. You can start small, simply throwing your board and some clothes in the car and heading down the coast. If you are thinking on a grander scale, it is hard to beat Hawaii. For surfers of every skill level, the Islands provide plenty of options, not to mention the birthplace of modern surfing (Waikiki) and the greatest show on surf (Oahu's North Shore during November/December). There is a wealth of travel information available on the Internet. Start with www.surfline.com and *Surfer Magazine's* "The Surf Report."

Take or rent – It is hard to imagine leaving your trusty friend at home, but traveling with surfboards can be a nightmare. A travel boardbag is a must and will cost anywhere from one hundred to a few hundred dollars. Airlines charge exorbitant fees (sometimes more than your board is worth) and often inflict damage along the way. On the other hand, you may not find rentals wherever you are going or they may be nothing like what you normally ride at home. Either way, it's rough.

Guided tour vs. solo mission – How much do you love adventure? If you consider yourself a fledgling Indiana Jones, or you simply cannot afford to pay for a guide, by all means do it yourself. A bit of difficulty on the road to success makes it that much sweeter when you discover it. If your eyes and mind remain open, you can find your way around. You might spend half your trip being lost, but you will have some great stories to tell. A guide, however, can prove invaluable. Knowing where to go, you will catch infinitely more waves.

Encountering localism – R-E-S-P-E-C-T, don't leave home without it. At most surf spots, the locals are not entirely opposed to visitors as long as those visitors are not greedy or otherwise rude. Wave hogs, loudmouths, and general kooks of any kind are despised everywhere. Take some time to learn the customs and be sure to leave your "Ugly American" side at home.

Learning the lay of the land – Whenever I visit a new place, I like to take a walk and get accustomed to my new surroundings. This gives me my bearings and prevents the possibility of getting lost later. Figure out the quickest route to the beach, the restaurant situation, and potential pitfalls such as prickly walkways or vicious neighborhood dogs.

All in the family? – There are family trips and there are surf trips. Unless the whole family surfs, taking the entire brood on a surf trip can be frustrating.

At some destinations, there is plenty for everyone to do—shopping, spas, pools, games, etc. However, many surf spots are located far from the beaten path. When you are not surfing, you are eating or swatting mosquitoes while napping before the next session. If you must bring the family, make sure your destination has family-friendly options.

Luck is where preparation meets opportunity – Every surfer has had a trip with absolutely no surf. Getting skunked happens to us all. You can increase your chances of scoring by doing your homework. Many destinations offer paradise one season followed by pure hell the next. Planning your trip to coincide with the best time for surf at a particular location is not always feasible. If you have that luxury, by all means exercise it. You are never guaranteed to catch epic surf, but you can certainly help your cause with due diligence.

CHAPTER 10 - SURFBOARDS 'R' US

In This Chapter

Anatomy of a Surfboard

Technical Elements of Design

Surfboard Evolution

Surfboard Construction

New vs. Used

Custom vs. Stock

Hard vs. Soft

Shortboard

Longboard

Funboard

Fish

Gun

Caring for Your Stick

CHAPTER 10 – SURFBOARDS "R" US

As legendary big wave pioneer Buzzy Trent famously said, "You don't go hunting elephant with a BB gun. If you're going to hunt big waves, take a big gun." Having the proper equipment for the surf conditions is paramount to success. Whether you are trying to stand up for the first time, grabbing a few waves after work, about to paddle out for a contest that will decide the world title, or staring out at the biggest waves of your life, there is a particular board for every situation. There are as many different models of surfboards as there are cars on the road. Each performs well under some conditions and not so well under others.

The question is, which one do you need?

Fortunately, as important as it is to pick the proper stick, choosing the right tool for the job is not too difficult. Many surfers acquire a quiver, or collection of boards in varying shapes and sizes. Once you understand how each board performs, the answer usually presents itself. Learning the nuances of a certain design can only take place in the water, so get out there and try as many different boards as you can. By doing so, you will figure out what works for you and what you like, which are usually the same thing.

"HEY, KOOK!" **You're not going to ride that, are you?**
I expect many readers ride either a funboard or a longboard. Unfortunately, there are conditions that preclude the use of these boards. When the waves are exceptionally hollow and/or powerful, a shortboard makes much more sense. Conversely, in waves that are small and weak, a longboard or fish makes the most sense.

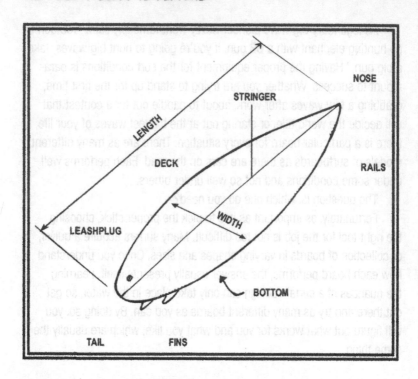

Anatomy of a Surfboard

Regardless of your chosen surfboard, it will possess each of the following features. In order to speak to other surfers in regards to boards, you should familiarize yourself with each of these terms.

Nose – The first twelve inches of a surfboard starting at the tip.

Tail – The last twelve inches of a surfboard starting from the tail.

Rails – The rounded perimeter or sides of a surfboard.

Deck – The mainly flat top part of a surfboard upon which a surfer stands.

Bottom – The underside of a surfboard.

Length – Measurement in feet and inches from the nose to the tail of a surfboard.

Width – Measurement in inches of a surfboard from rail to rail at its wide point.

Thickness – Measurement in inches from deck to bottom at the thickest part of a surfboard.

Fins – Device (or devices) along the underside of a surfboard that serve as rudders. They aid in drive, direction, and control of the surfboard. Typically curved in the shape of a dolphin's dorsal fin. Can either be permanently fixed to the board with fiberglass or attached via a fin box.

Leash plug – A small plug typically placed in the deck near the tail of a surfboard used to attach a leash.

Stringer – A narrow wooden strip along the vertical center of a surfboard that adds strength.

Technical Elements of Design

Outline – The template, or defining shape of a surfboard. Established by measuring the width of a board at established intervals, primarily 12" from the tip, at the wide point (close to, but not necessary at, the midpoint), and 12" from the tail.

Template – A wooden pattern used by a shaper to draw the surfboard's outline on a blank prior to shaping. Typically made of thin plywood, plastic, or Masonite. Shapers usually create templates from existing boards and keep them in their shaping room for future use.

Foil – The rate of change of a surfboard's thickness from the nose to the tail, also of a surfboard fin.

Rocker – The amount of curve along the bottom of a surfboard from nose to tail as viewed from the side. This controls the flow of water beneath a board and thus greatly affects speed and maneuverability.

(More rocker=more curve=slower and easier to turn. Less rocker=less curve=faster and more difficult to turn.)

Bottom contours – Design features along the underside of a surfboard that impact its speed and maneuverability, including concaves, channels, and vee.

Drag – More of an effect than a particular design element. Drag, or water resistance, helps with control, making this a necessary feature in the design of a surfboard.

Drive – The ability of a surfboard to accelerate along a wave. This effect is created by water pressure against a surface.

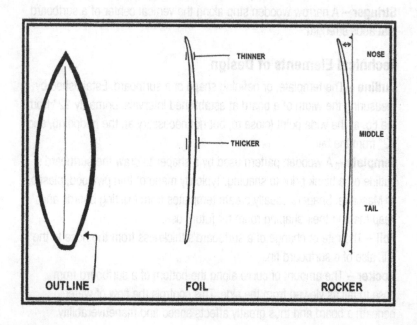

OUTLINE   FOIL   ROCKER

Surfboard Evolution

Carrying a rider along a wave is the only thing modern surfboards have in common with those used by Polynesians and Hawaiians a thousand years ago. There aren't many people in the world today that could ride an ancient board with any degree of success. To say we have it easy is an understatement. We are spoiled rotten.

The early Hawaiian surfboards were little more than flat planks of solid wood with crudely pointed or rounded noses. They measured anywhere from a few feet ("paipo" boards, sort of an ancient boogie board), to around ten feet ("alaia" boards ridden by commoners), to sixteen or more feet in length ("olo" boards reserved exclusively for royalty). The longer models, as you might imagine, were terribly cumbersome and weighed as much as 200 pounds.

These ancient boards remained in use until after surfing was rediscovered in the twentieth century. Tom Blake, among the sport's guiding lights, created a much lighter, "hollow" board during the 1920's and followed up by introducing the fin the following decade. "Hot Curls" came along around the same time, featuring a narrowed tail to allow more maneuverability and holding power in larger surf. This allowed surfers to ride parallel to the wave rather than straight in. Balsa offered a further reduction in weight during the 1940's, cutting the burden in half to around 40 pounds.

Technology created during World War II instigated the greatest changes to surfboard development. After the war, board builders began experimenting with foam and fiberglass, and by the late '50s the process was perfected. Surfboards, all of a sudden, became far easier to mass-produce and market. The surfing population swelled as a result, and surf shops sprouted up and down both coasts of the United States. A typical board in the early '60s was close to ten feet in length, around

23" wide, and sported a single large, boxy fin. Change was right around the corner, and these relics soon would come to be known as "classic longboards."

In 1968, The Beatles tore into the blitzing opening chords of "Revolution." John Lennon promised that it was "gonna be all right," but for longboards the end had already begun. During the "shortboard revolution," shapers drastically reduced the length of boards in order to obtain increased maneuverability. No longer content to merely ride a wave, surfers sought to explore its every nook and cranny. Within a couple years, a six-foot board became standard issue for this so-called "involvement" surfing. Throughout the '70s there was a time of experimentation during which many ideas failed miserably. In 1981, however, Australian pro surfer/shaper Simon Anderson hit on the three-fin Thruster concept, a design that remains in common use today.

While the thruster continues to dictate performance standards, surfers have grown nostalgic and brought several old ideas back into the mix. Longboards resurfaced during the 1990s, and the fish design of the '70s has gained widespread popularity. Nowadays, it is common to see boards from every era, including replicas of ancient Hawaiian planks, all sharing the same lineup.

Surfboard Construction

Many hours of labor go into creating a handmade surfboard. Since boards have become so easy to come by, a miniscule percentage of surfers ever undertake shaping, glassing, and sanding their own board. The process can be grueling, intense, and nasty enough to land on the Discovery Channel show *Dirty Jobs* (season one, episode nine). Most choose to leave boardbuilding to the professionals.

A surfboard begins as a dense polyurethane slab known as a "blank." These blanks are blown using molds and can be obtained in various sizes, shapes, and strengths. The first person to touch the blank is the most crucial, the shaper. These days, the majority of boards are crafted using a shaping machine, and the shaper merely fine-tunes to achieve a finished product. Some shapers still do it all by hand, either refusing to succumb to the technological revolution or because they cannot afford to. The shaper uses a template to pencil an outline on the blank. With a handsaw, he then cuts along the outline. A planer is the main tool of a shaper, used to mill the blank to the preferred thickness. A respirator, goggles, and earplugs are worn for safety. Finally, he spends a considerable amount of time fine-tuning every inch of the blank to achieve the desired design. The entire shaping process takes roughly two hours per board.

Glassing, or laminating, the finished blank with a protective coat of fiberglass is the next step in the process. This procedure is accomplished one side at a time. First the bottom, and once that dries for about a day, then the deck. Each side is covered with a thin, woven sheet of fiberglass cloth and a bucket of syrup-y resin that is applied with a squeegee. Fin boxes are installed next, followed by another thinner layer of resin, known as the "hot coat."

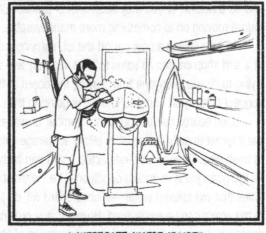

A SURFBOARD SHAPER AT WORK.

Sanding the surfboard will then remove any imperfections and leave the glass job smooth and shiny. After a few days of curing, the surfboard is ready for the water.

New vs. Used

If you have never been on a surfboard, there are multiple reasons for not starting your surfing life on a new board. First, you never know for sure if you will continue surfing, so purchasing a board off the racks could be a colossal waste of money. (I cannot see how anyone would decide that one time on a surfboard is enough, but it happens. Plenty of people start out with a single miserable session and retire their sea legs forever.) Another reason not to start on a new board is that your chances of ruining it are greatest while you are at your kookiest. In the beginning, you have not learned to fall gracefully, and an elbow or knee through the deck makes for a serious bummer. And finally, until you ride a few waves, you cannot know for certain what board will best work for you. You might surprise yourself and be a natural, or you may need a lot of practice on a beginner board before moving on to something more maneuverable.

As with driving a new car off the lot, carrying a surfboard out the door of a surf shop causes its value to drop instantly and significantly. I am not trying to dissuade anyone from buying the board of their dreams, but I suggest holding off until you know it is going to be a good fit.

Used boards can be found in a number of places, from surf shops, to the Internet (mainly Craigslist or eBay), to garage sales, and occasionally in trash bins. Often, a long-neglected board can be had for a song. As long as the glass job is in decent condition—i.e., without an overabundance of holes that will take on water—a used board will do just fine. A few chinks in the armor can be easily fixed. However, any prolonged water seepage eventually leads to de-lamination, or separation of fiberglass from foam, a difficult and costly dilemma. Give a used board a thorough examination before buying it. If you give the rail a squeeze and water gushes out like a geyser, this is probably not a match made in heaven.

Custom vs. Stock

In our modern society of instant gratification, the surfboard industry has come along for the ride. With computer-generated shapes, pop-outs from Asia, and catalogs of pre-dimensioned point-and-purchase models, the custom surfboard seems well on its way to following the fate of the dodo bird. Some long-time surfers lament this transformation, but if you can get exactly what you want without waiting two months (the average return time on a custom board), then the change sounds like progress to me.

Still, there is plenty to be said for ordering, and patiently waiting for, a one-of-a-kind custom stick. I order each of my boards from my trusty shaper. Not only does the process hearken back to a time when surfing was still an individual, rebellious endeavor, but the feeling of finally getting that phone call and rushing down to the surf shop to lay eyes on your new love is priceless. I imagine this is sort of like sending away for a mail-order bride. You wait and wait, and as soon as she lands at the airport, you are high-tailing it down to meet her.

Surfboard shaping used to be an esteemed career path for an avid surfer. In fact, other than a few guys getting paid to perform surf demonstrations or lessons for tourists, shaping was the first career in surfing. Skyrocketing costs and overseas competition have all but pushed the small-time boardbuilder out of business. It is still possible to order a custom surfboard, and I would highly recommend doing so. It might take some searching, so poke around at your local surf shop or in the lineup for some potential shapers. Whatever you do, when you find a shaper, be honest with him in regards to your abilities. Do not tell him you are a hero when your wave count is usually zero. Tell him the truth and trust in his skills to build you a soul mate.

Hard vs. Soft

Choosing between a hard fiberglass board and one that is covered with soft foam comes down to one simple question: How serious are you about surfing? Foam boards are wonderful for learning how to catch waves and stand up. If you fall and the board hits you, it does not hurt (that much). This is the reason surf camps use softboards almost exclusively. They are ideal for learning the basics and especially for young children. If surfing, for you, is something you plan to do only a handful of times per year, then buying a soft board might be a good idea. A good softboard will withstand much abuse and is not prone to cracks and dings every time

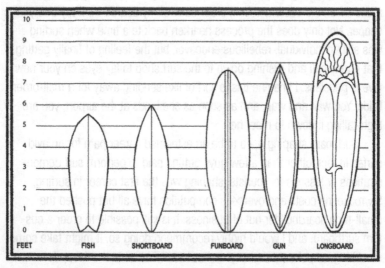

you drop it on the way to the beach. Beyond that, softboards are extremely limited in their performance capabilities. They tend to be blockier and less fine-tuned, somewhat similar to a surfboard blank before it is shaped. Therefore, softboards have difficultly turning and generating down-the-line speed. If you expect to surf a lot and hope to progress, I suggest going with a fiberglass board.

Shortboard

The performance thruster has been the standard shortboard since 1981. These three-finned potato chips look easy enough to ride when you see someone who knows what he is doing, but in reality, they are extremely difficult, especially in small surf. They are not particularly adept at paddling or catching waves, and while on a wave the surfer must pump the board from rail to rail just to keep from sinking. Furthermore, short-boards can be overly sensitive and make an unbalanced rider look as if he is having a seizure. If maneuvers are what you are after, you will overlook the shortboard's drawbacks and figure out how to make it work.

Experience Needed: Intermediate/ Expert

Average Length: Around 6'0", but can go much shorter for small kids or longer for larger people

Average Width: 18"–19"

Average Thickness: 2.2"–2.75"

Rocker: Full

Fins: Three

Weight: Light

Paddling/Wave Catching Ease: Low

Duck Diving Ease: High

Speed: Low

Maneuverability: High

Ideal Conditions: Waist-high to double-overhead

Longboard

If a smooth ride is your cup of tea, these classic boards from surfing's days of yore make riding waves as easy as walking down the sidewalk. A longboard is a valuable addition to any quiver and can turn a tiny summer day into a boatload of fun. Longboards make paddling, catching waves, standing, and balancing a breeze. Seeing a true Old School longboarder in action is a pleasure to watch, his entire ride a seamless, flowing masterpiece. Then again, when I see a kook who could not otherwise catch a single wave hogging a lineup because he is atop one of these paddling machines, I want to puke.

Experience Needed: Beginner/Intermediate
Average Length: 9'–10'
Average Width: 22"–23"
Average Thickness: 2.4"–3"
Rocker: Slight
Fins: One for classic styling, three for "progressive" maneuvering

Weight: Heavy
Paddling/Wave Catching Ease: High
Duck Diving Ease: Low
Speed: High
Maneuverability: Low
Ideal Conditions: Ankle to head-high

Funboard

These "mid-range" boards came of age during the late '80s surfing revival and attracted former surfers disenfranchised with shortboards back to the water. Nowadays, funboards are generally ridden either by middle-agers who want more maneuverability than a longboard provides or by youngsters new to the sport.

Experience Needed: Beginner/
Intermediate
Average Length: 7'6"–8'10"
Average Width: 20"–22"
Average Thickness: 2.5"–3"
Rocker: Moderate
Fins: Three
Weight: Moderate

Paddling/Wave Catching Ease:
High
Duck Diving Ease: Low
Speed: Moderate
Maneuverability: Moderate
Ideal Conditions: Knee-high to
slightly overhead

Fish

Designed in the early '70s for kneeboarders and stand-up surfers to ride tighter to the curl, these speed demons disappeared for two decades before thankfully re-emerging. They make a good starter board for an aggressive kid, but their resurgence is due to folks tired of sinking in small waves on traditional shortboards. These stumpy twin-fins are amazingly fast down the line but must be maneuvered gingerly to keep from losing control.

Experience Needed: Intermediate
Average Length: 5'6"–6'6"
Average Width: 19.5"–21.5"
Average Thickness: 2.25"–2.75"
Rocker: Slight
Fins: Two
Weight: Light
Paddling/Wave Catching Ease:
High

Duck Diving Ease: Moderate
Speed: High
Maneuverability: Moderate, prone
to sliding out
Ideal Conditions: Knee-high to
slightly overhead

Gun

Developed during the early days of big wave surfing along Oahu's North and West shores, these sleek beauties are built for survival. Guns are used for paddle surfing as opposed to tow-ins (watercraft-assisted surfing) because they provide ample paddling ability at the expense of maneuverability. They have a large amount of rocker in order to negotiate steep drops.

Experience Needed: Expert

Average Length: 6'8"–10'0", depending on the surf

Average Width: 18.5"–19.5"

Average Thickness: 2.25"–2.75"

Rocker: Extreme

Fins: Three, rarely one

Weight: Light/moderate

Paddling/Wave Catching Ease: High

Duck Diving Ease: Moderate

Speed: Low

Maneuverability: Moderate

Ideal Conditions: Double-over-head plus

Caring for your Stick

Surfboards are fragile, but their lives can be extended with proper care. A mistreated stick, on the other hand, will rapidly lose its spark and eventually fall apart beneath your feet. Therefore, be proactive. The best investment you can make to keep your board in ship shape is a boardbag. There are expensive travel bags (thick, sturdy, and roomy for air travel), less expensive day bags (thinner and not so roomy for general daily use), and el-cheapo board socks (soft and snug-fitting like the name implies). At the least, invest twenty-or-so bucks in a board sock to prevent discoloration from sun exposure and provide a minimal amount of padding.

Exercise care when transporting your board, whether taking it around the world, putting it in the car, or toting it down the street on your bike. When using a travel bag, removing the fins and wrapping the board in bubble wrap or some other padding in addition to the bag is a good idea. Better safe than sorry, as nothing ruins a week in paradise faster than arriving with a broken stick. (For air travel, also know that the airlines charge around a hundred dollars or more for each surfboard bag. Some particularly ornery agents have been known to open a board bag and charge a fee for each board inside.) A roof rack is suggested for automobile travel, as it protects your board and your car's interior. Racks run the gamut from high-tech hard racks to simple nylon straps. Any surf shop will be happy to install the rack and show you the right way to use it. If you live close enough to the beach to pedal, a bicycle rack will free your hands up for steering and waving to girls.

The newer your board looks, the more likely you are to take care of it. Therefore, occasionally cleaning the wax and applying a fresh coat has been known to renew an old love affair. Take care of your board on land, and it will take care of you in the water.

CHAPTER 11 - SURF STUFF

In This Chapter
Bathing Suit
Wetsuit
Fins
Wax
Leash
Random and Not-So-Random Accessories

Compared to many athletic endeavors, surfing requires little in the way of equipment aside from a single necessity—a surfboard. Sure, you need a wave, but unfortunately Mother Nature cannot be bought or even persuaded. You may be waiting a while for the fickle old broad to send something your way, but with a board at least you are ready. If you are a frugal and diligent shopper, and unafraid of sporting a stick that has seen better days, you can be in the water for under a hundred bucks. There are, however, several other items that can make your surfing experience easier and more enjoyable. Some are necessary, while others might be considered luxury items or even downright useless. It is up to you to decide what you take to the beach.

Bathing Suit

Many ancient Hawaiians surfed in nothing but the fresh salt air and the sweet smell of plumeria—i.e., naked. Loincloths gained favor in the 1800s, followed by woolen tank suits to start the next century. When surfing began to grow, people wore whatever shorts they could find. It was not until the 1950s that some California transplants on Oahu went to a local tailor for custom-made "surf trunks." These precursors of the modern boardshort came complete with a stripe down the side and a wax pocket. By the early '60s, California companies Katin and Hang Ten were making and selling large quantities of nylon surf trunks. Manufacturers began popping up all over to satisfy the demand for boardshorts, and the surf clothing industry was born.

Modern boardshorts are not too different from those produced decades ago. Sure, they are longer now, but they are essentially the same bright, Velcro-fly, nylon shorts with a pocket for carrying surf wax. Despite the advancements in technology, they will still give you a hellacious rash when you wear them every day for a week straight.

Not to be outdone, female surfers got their own surf trunks in the early '90s when Quiksilver began producing a line called Roxy. Their attractive world champion surfer Lisa Andersen sported the snug-fitting shorts around the globe, and a mega fashion trend soon followed.

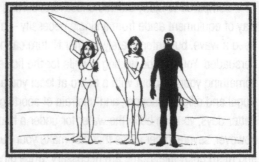

FROM BIKINIS, TO SPRINGSUITS, TO FULL RUBBER ARMOR, SURFERS ARE FOUND IN VARIOUS STATES OF DRESS.

Boardshorts are designed specifically for surfing. They stretch where they need to be stretchy, breathe where they need to be breathable, and stay on when you need them to stay on. But do you really need to wear "boardshorts" to be a surfer? Absolutely not. Wearing the latest $75 surf company boardshorts will not keep you from being a kook, but they might make the fact a little harder to recognize, at least until you hit the water.

Wetsuit

I cannot tell you how many times I have been stopped en route to a winter surf by an elderly female tourist who just has to know, "Do those things really keep you warm?" Yes, Grandma, wetsuits indeed serve a purpose aside from making us look like superheroes. They also keep us warm. And unless you reside in the tropics, you will eventually need a wetsuit if you wish to keep surfing.

Wetsuits come in various thicknesses (measured in millimeters) and designs. You have your vest, your short-sleeve jacket, your long-sleeve jacket, your short john (think high school wrestling uniform), your long john (wrestling uniform top with long legs, a design that has thankfully gone extinct), your short-sleeve spring suit (short arm/short leg), your long-sleeve spring suit, your short-sleeve full suit, and, finally, your long-sleeve full suit. Which one you need depends on the water temperature. Seventy-five and up, you are good with just a bathing suit. Upper sixties to low seventies call for a spring suit. Anything in the low sixties or below, a full suit is in order. Once you dip into the fifties, you're talking boots and even gloves and a hood. In the forties, nothing should be exposed to the elements but your face.

Technology in regards to wetsuits has been nothing short of amazing over the last couple decades. Even in water that hovers around the freezing mark, this body armor not only fights off hypothermia, it can make you almost comfortable. We owe our wonderful warmth to a man named Jack O'Neill who grew tired of freezing his nuts off in the chilly water at Santa Cruz. In the early '50s, Jack stumbled upon a new material known as neoprene and fashioned a tight-fitting bodysuit from it. A half-century later, O'Neill is the most respected name in wetsuits. Thanks to Jack, surfing has spread far beyond the tropics to nearly every place on earth with a coastline.

Contrary to what you might think, wetsuits do not keep a surfer dry. (That would be a drysuit, an air-tight, loose-fitting nylon suit that used to be worn by surfers in the Northeast before wetsuits drastically improved.) Wetsuits fit snug to your skin but allow a thin layer of seawater to penetrate. Your body warms that water, which then acts as insulation.

Wetsuit care includes rinsing it in fresh water after each use and hanging it to dry. Try not to leave it roasting in the sun or balled up in a wet heap on the floor. Also, resist the temptation to toss your suit in the dryer. While it sucks to have to put on a cold suit, the dryer will break down the glue that holds together the seams. When you are finished with your suit for the year, be sure to give it a thorough rinse and dry and store it somewhere free of mildew.

Fins

You either like a surfboard or you don't. A board does not have a bunch of interchangeable parts that substantially alter the way it performs. One exception is fins, assuming they are of the exchangeable variety rather than permanently fixed with fiberglass. (In that case, you are completely out of luck.) Fins are often overlooked in terms of importance, yet they can sometimes turn a lazy dog of a board into a greyhound.

Fins affect the drive, maneuverability, and holding power of the surfboard. The smaller the fins, the slower a board will ride down-the-line and the more sensitive it will be under applied pressure. With larger fins, a board will assume more down-the-line drive but become stiffer through turns. It is this interplay of drive and stiffness that often determines how well a board works. Spending some time trying out various fin setups should prove a worthwhile endeavor.

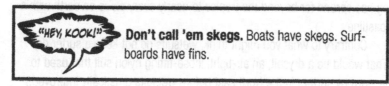

"HEY, KOOK!" **Don't call 'em skegs.** Boats have skegs. Surfboards have fins.

Wax

Aside from waves and a board, wax is the third most crucial component to going surfing. Wax provides traction between your body and the deck while paddling, and between your feet and the deck when standing. Sure, this sticky, gooey mass has been known to wreak havoc on car interiors, clothes dryers (when you forget to remove it from your pocket), and chest hair, but it comes in quite handy when trying to stay atop a surfboard. No wax, and you are likely performing a split on takeoff.

There are several brands of surf wax on the market, and any real surf shop carries plenty of choices for around a buck a bar. On the wrapper, you will find information detailing the conditions for which that particular formula is designed. Cold water wax is the softest of the bunch so it will keep from freezing under your feet in frigid surroundings. Cool water wax is slightly harder, followed by warm water wax, and finally tropical, the hardest consistency in order to prevent melting.

A thorough coat of wax should be applied to the deck of a new surfboard prior to use. This process should take about five minutes and use around a half-bar of wax. In general, you want to cover the lower two-thirds of the deck spreading out to where the rails begin to curve downward. Press the wax against the deck and give it a thorough covering. For subsequent sessions, a quick once-over with the wax is all that is necessary. To protect a wax job, never leave your board "deck up" toward the sun or plop it "deck down" in the sand. Either will quickly ruin your traction. Eventually, through frequent use, your wax job will turn a filthy shade of brown. When that happens, it is time to strip off the old wax and start again from scratch.

A wax comb is a multi-faceted tool used to remove old surf wax as well as to rough up a wax job for increased traction. Many new pairs of boardshorts come with a wax comb in the pocket. As a kid, I used my mom's spatula for removing old wax. It worked great, but for some reason she was not as happy about that fact as I was. Maybe I should have cleaned the spatula afterwards. I suggest leaving the kitchen utensils in their place and getting a comb.

The radical brand of shortboard surfing that emerged in the 1970s and early '80s led some to look for a stickier alternative to surf wax. Thus, the traction pad was born. There are several companies manufacturing these foam rubber stick-on pads in a plethora of textures and color schemes. Most bear the name and signature of this or that pro surfer and will set you back around thirty bucks. The pads adhere to the rear section of the deck and keep the back foot firmly planted in place. Particularly for shortboards, traction pads are a good idea.

"HEY, KOOK!" **Get that wax out of your mouth.** Please use the pocket in your trunks if you need to take some wax with you into the water. When someone paddles out with a bar of wax clenched in his teeth, he reminds me of a roasted pig at a luau with an apple stuffed in its mouth.

Leash

The surf leash is a safety mechanism that keeps a rider from becoming separated from his surfboard. This thin urethane strap measures around six feet in length and connects from the leash plug at the rear of the surfboard to a surfer's ankle. For about twenty dollars, it not only protects you from being stranded in the lineup as your board smashes into a pier or some rocks, it also keeps your runaway stick from turning into a deadly projectile that might harm another surfer.

Leashes came into existence in the early 1970s when shorter boards and aggressive maneuvering led to more wipeouts. Early leashes were extremely stretchy—often using a bungee cord, putting the rider in a precarious situation as he emerged from a wipeout only to find his board snapping back at him. Since beginners tend to fall more regularly than experienced surfers, leashes quickly earned the unfavorable moniker of "kook cords." The stigma soon evaporated as more surfers flocked toward this safety net.

Modern surf leashes are constructed of sturdy but flexible urethane. They come in various lengths and thicknesses to match a rider's board size and the surf conditions. A six-foot leash is good for a shortboard, while an eight- or ten-footer makes sense with a longboard or gun. To fasten a leash, tie one end to your leash plug and strap the Velcro tether around the ankle on your back leg (right ankle for a regularfoot; left for a goofyfoot). Metal swivels at either end help keep the leash from getting twisted. Most leashes also have a "rail saver" that prevents the cord from pulling through the tail of the board during a wipeout.

Leashes have had a major impact on surfing. On one hand, the invention helped expand performance levels by eliminating lengthy swims after wipeouts. It is much easier to push the limits when you know your board will be waiting for you if you take a spill. On the other hand, our dependence on the leash has made modern surfers lazier than previous generations. These safety straps have eliminated our need to become true watermen.

"HEY, KOOK!" **Unstrap the leash when you get out of the water.** Do not wait until you get to your car to unstrap it. The odds of a tsunami hitting you in the parking lot are slim to none.

Random and Not-So-Random Accessories

Surf Bin – If you find yourself turning into a surfer, your health and happiness may be on the upswing, but before long your car will definitely suffer. Sand, surf wax, and mildewed wetsuits quickly turn your sweet ride into a stink-mobile. Not to worry, this dilemma can be cured with the help of a sealable, five-dollar storage bin that will live in the back of the car. A bin is ideal for keeping your messy and smelly accessories contained. Plus, you will always know where to find the sunscreen, spare fins, or any other easily misplaced surf paraphernalia.

Sunscreen – Always be sure to lather up with a non-greasy, waterproof sunscreen prior to entering the water. You will get tan whether you want to or not, but sunburns can be prevented.

Rashguard – A Lycra surf shirt serves multiple purposes. First, as the name implies, a rashguard keeps one's chest and stomach from getting rubbed raw from the deck of a surfboard. It can also be worn underneath a wetsuit that chafes around the neck or armpits. Additionally, a rashguard provides a layer of protection from sun exposure.

Earplugs – For some surfers, prolonged exposure to the elements can cause problems with the ear canal and hearing. Earplugs can prevent water and wind from entering the ear canal. Companies such as Doc's Pro-plugs sell earplugs designed specifically for surfing.

Belly Jelly – When it comes to preventing or treating a rash from a surfboard or wetsuit, Belly Jelly or some other aloe-based gel does the trick. Vaseline also serves as a rash preventative.

Surf Hat – As the dangers of sun exposure become more widely known, increasing numbers of surfers are donning wide-brimmed hats in the water. Typically affixed with a chin-strap for security, a surf hat can also cut down on glare. I have heard it said that only kooks surf in hats. Considering that I rarely surf without one during the summer, I am not buying into that nonsense.

Noseguard – The nose on a surfboard, especially a pointy one, can be a dangerous weapon. No one will call you a kook for sticking a rubber tip on the front of your stick for safety purposes. Produced by NoseGuard Hawaii and sold for just over ten dollars, they might save your eye one day.

Webbed Gloves – These snazzy little mitts were rolled out along with big hair and day-glo in the 1980s, and that is where they should have stayed. Sure, they might provide the wearer with a touch more propulsion with each stroke, but the kook factor is through the roof.

Water Shoes –
Wearing booties in cold water or even reef walkers for traversing razor-sharp coral are one thing. Protecting one's tootsies from a potential crab pinch or brush up against "eww-ee" seaweed with water

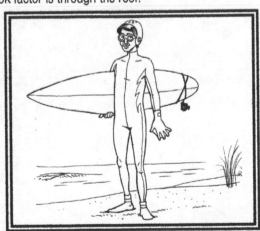

shoes is quite another. Unless you are a foot model, do not even think about it.

> **"HEY, KOOK!"** **Lose the mittens and bath slippers.**
> Webbed gloves and water shoes are made for
> kooks, pure and simple.

PART IV: MANEUVERS

CHAPTER 12 - A FOUNDATION FOR HIGHER LEARNING

In This Chapter

CHAPTER 12 – A FOUNDATION FOR HIGHER LEARNING

In This Chapter

Mind Surfing

Wave Selection and Lineup Positioning

Get in the Pocket

Generating Speed

Style

Bigger and Better Things

Tips for Further Improvement

Do not even think about skipping ahead to the next chapter without thoroughly ingesting this one first. This is the most important section in this book, possibly the most crucial words your eyes will ever read. It is all here in black and white, the ancient and previously unpublished keys to successful surfing. *The Da Vinci Code,* the lost city of Atlantis, who shot JFK?—those mysteries are child's play compared to the top-secret information you are about to receive! Without the knowledge in this chapter, you are doomed to live out your surfing days in a pitiful state of perpetual kookdom. Without acquiring these essential building blocks, your surfing will sink like the *Titanic.*

Mind Surfing

All thoughts seem to disappear the instant a surfer catches a wave; yet, I would hardly consider surfing a mindless pursuit. In fact, when considering tools for improvement, a mind is a terrible thing to waste. Mind surfing involves sitting on the beach and imagining yourself riding a wave as you watch it break. Whether the surf is two inches or twenty feet, perfectly peeling or hopelessly closing out, anyone with half an imagination can rip a wave in this make-believe world. Not only is it fun, I regard mind surfing as extremely helpful.

Visualization has gradually gained acceptance as a tool for performance enhancement throughout sports as well as in the workplace and in daily life. The concept is simple: Imagine yourself succeeding, and the odds of that happening improve. You have to admit that the mere idea of riding waves, not to mention simultaneously performing acrobatic maneuvers atop a slender strip of foam without falling off, sounds preposterous. Seeing it happen in one's mind makes the prospect easier to digest.

After decades of surfing and mind surfing, I am physically unable to look at a wave and not imagine myself riding it. And in my mind, I am a far better surfer than in real life. We all are. I can pull off every trick in the book, and I never fall. For added impact, I use my hand to represent my surfboard and even throw in some slashing sound effects.

As you begin to mind surf, avoid giving your avatar freaky, cartoon-ish abilities. He should be better than you, but not that much better. First imagine successfully riding a wave from start to finish. Try to pinpoint the ideal takeoff spot to begin your imaginary ride. From there, simply keep your make-believe self in the steepest and best-shaped part of the wave. Once you can perform this feat with reasonable success in real life, you can expand your horizons. Your mind surfing will always remain one step ahead of the actual you.

Wave Selection and Lineup Positioning

A big part of gaining proficiency at surfing comes from learning to catch better waves. Ninety-nine percent of the time, catching good waves has nothing to do with luck. If you watch a crowded surf session, you will notice the same few surfers in position ("on-the-button") for all the best waves. Sure, some kook will accidently wander into the perfect spot on occasion, but that situation is rare. The question is, What do those surfers on-the-button know that you don't?

For one thing, they are observant. Before they set foot in the water, they have already scoped out the situation and determined the location of the ideal take-off spot. To do this, they watch a few sets roll through and get a fix on where the waves initially break. They pinpoint an area just outside of the peak and paddle towards it. Once in the lineup, they go to that mark and wait for a set. If they find themselves slightly out of position when a set arrives, they take note and re-establish themselves in the correct spot.

In order to be on-the-button, it is best to set up camp roughly ten to twenty feet directly beyond where you plan to drop into a wave. That distance provides a runway of sorts to build paddling speed prior to liftoff. You want to be cruising down the wave face when it is steepening but not yet beginning to break. Doing so allows enough time to stand and get to the bottom of the wave before the lip begins to topple. Accomplishing this feat requires practice and plenty of mishaps. To gauge whether or not you are in the spot, take a look at the wave over your shoulder while paddling. You might need to either speed up your paddling if the wave is reluctant to break or slow it down if the lip is already pitching. Learn from any mistakes and in time you will be on-the-button more often than not.

"HEY, KOOK!"

Know your surroundings. Do not paddle out and let the ocean have its way with you. Pick a spot to sit and stay there. If you have to paddle against a steady current, do it. You will get into surf shape that much faster.

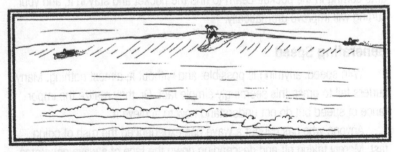

THE SURFER TO THE LEFT IS TOO FAR INSIDE, THE ONE ON THE RIGHT TOO FAR OUT, AND
THE ONE IN THE MIDDLE IS JUST RIGHT.

Get in the Pocket

No, we are not talking about billiards. Just as there is an ideal spot to catch a wave, there is an area on every wave that best lends itself to surfing. That area is known as the "pocket." Located on the steep part of the wave face just ahead of the whitewater, the pocket moves down-the-line along with the breaking wave. The steepness continually propels the rider along the wave and provides the optimal sections for performing maneuvers. Behind the pocket, a surfer becomes stuck in the whitewater and unable to maneuver, while the area ahead of the pocket may not be steep enough to keep him moving.

The ability to consistently surf in the pocket represents a major stepping-stone in the education process. Interestingly, doing so often requires learning to do nothing as much as doing something. In our haste to "make" a wave, it is easy to get so far ahead of the pocket that we leave our energy source and end up losing the wave. Whenever you find yourself running out of steam on the shoulder, the best remedy is straightening out and waiting for the pocket to catch up. If you watch the best surfers in the lineup (and in the world), you will notice that they spend most or all of their time surfing in the pocket. Learn to find the pocket and stay in it, and your surfing will improve dramatically.

Generating Speed

With speed, anything is possible, and without it, almost nothing. Many surfers fail to grasp this seemingly simple fact. Or, they realize the importance of speed but do not understand how to achieve it.

Anyone who has caught a wave has experienced the rush of going fast. Merely taking off and descending down the face of a wave generates velocity. Unfortunately, that speed quickly dissipates once you reach the flat area at the bottom. Down-the-line momentum is another story. The key to building down-the-line speed is using the wave's incline and allowing gravity to work for you. By heading down the wave at an angle as opposed to straight toward the shore, it is possible to be riding down a perpetual incline. Therefore, speed is more easily maintained. Finding that sweet spot on the wave and locking into it is known as "trimming." A good bit of speed can be had by simply standing there once you locate the perfect position on the wave.

In order to perform many of today's high-flying maneuvers, an additional burst of speed is required. To generate even more velocity, surfers pump their board down-the-line. With pumping, a surfer squeezes every drop of speed from an incline by applying added pressure with the front foot. Upon reaching the bottom, lift the board back up the wave face and again jam it back down another incline. At the same time, alternate pressure between the heel-side and toe-side of the board to better facilitate the up-and-down movement. Repeating this process in rapid succession—when performed properly—can create vast amounts of speed.

There are two keys to successful pumping. The first is alternating pressure from rail to rail, smoothly shifting weight from toe-side to heel-side and back, rather than flapping up and down. "S-turning" or "roller coastering," as it is also known, can be easily practiced using a longboard skateboard on land before hitting the water.

The second important factor in pumping is learning to read the wave and take what it is willing to give. Pumping should not be executed willy-nilly, so do not force it! As a wave passes over varying bottom contours, it will speed up or slow down. Any wave, no matter how small, contains pockets with more energy than other sections of the wave. Finding these power pockets, and using their energy to generate speed, is the difference between flowing and flailing.

"HEY, KOOK!"

Quit killing the fish. When executed improperly, as it often is, pumping becomes a truly gruesome sight. I have witnessed countless surfers jumping around like spider monkeys and smacking their board against the wave in a fruitless search for speed. It looks as if they are attempting to murder an entire school of fish rather than merely trying to go fast. Little do they know that they could go much faster just by standing in the pocket and letting gravity run its course.

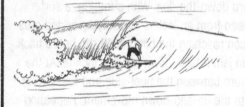

WHEN YOU LEARN TO RIDE IN THE POCKET, THE WAVE DOES MOST OF THE WORK FOR YOU.

Style

I could fill volumes trying to explain the concept of style in surfing, but I won't. I have been an avid student of style since I first stood on a surfboard, yet I hardly claim to be an expert on the matter. I have been told that I have "good style" when surfing, but any judgment on surf style is just that, a judgment call. Different strokes for different folks, as they say. What I do know about style is this: Good surfers make difficult moves look easy, and bad surfers make easy moves look more difficult than they are.

Everyone naturally develops his or her own surfing style. The way they hold their hands, the way their back hunches, the degree to which their limbs move—style is the combination of these traits and others. Sitting several blocks away, I can watch someone at my local break ride a wave and know instantly who it is just by his style. Our approach to riding waves probably says a lot about the kind of people we are on land. Are we overly aggressive or totally laid back, in a hurry or casually cool, creative or boring? The truth, I believe, comes out in the water.

Can we change our style? Yes, but it takes work. Altering the way we surf is possible, but doing so requires a concerted effort. When I was fourteen, I first saw a video of Tom Curren riding a wave at his home break in Santa Barbara, and I immediately re-examined my entire life, or at least my approach to surfing. Tom, the son of big-wave pioneer Pat Curren, emerged in the early '80s as America's best hope for a world title and a veritable style god. His entire body remained in sync at all times, and he never appeared out of control. Along with countless other teenaged surfers, I studied videos of Curren at every opportunity. I mimicked his style while skateboarding in front of my house and even while standing in front of the mirror. I will admit, it sounds kinda ridiculous, but to me, style mattered.

If style matters to you, find someone to film videos of you surfing. Until you see yourself on screen, you really cannot know how you surf. The important thing to watch is whether or not you flow with the wave. Does your style look more like Fred Astaire on the dance floor or a little brat throwing a tantrum in the check-out line at Wal-Mart? Do your limbs seem to work in unison or fling randomly like the tentacles on Doc Occ's back? Whatever the case, video provides the definitive answer.

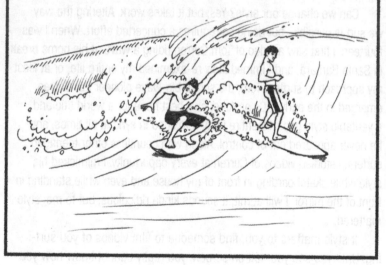

"HEY, KOOK!" **Keep your body under control.** It makes my stomach turn when I see kooks flailing their arms on a wave as if they are trying to get someone's attention on the beach. They think they are performing moves, but their board is usually not turning. Only their bodies are moving. Either get some outside advice or watch yourself on video. Otherwise, you might be surfing like a monkey.

TOO MUCH BODY MOVEMENT CAN BE COUNTERPRODUCTIVE. SOMETIMES IT'S BETTER TO JUST STAND THERE.

Bigger and Better Things

Every surfer at one time finds himself standing on the sand, board in arm, struggling to make a decision—to go or not to go. He stares out at waves that are bigger than anything he has ever experienced, and the butterflies in his gut are flapping like mad. My advice is to be smart about the situation by considering the worst-case scenario. Graduating to larger surf should be incremental. Do not rush into waves that are exponentially larger than what you have ridden. If you paddle out, be ready to have a set of waves on your head. If after studying the lineup you feel confident that you can survive being caught in the impact zone without much worry, then go for it.

One important consideration before taking such a leap is your level of fitness. The bigger the surf, the more critical fitness becomes. Energy expenditure increases dramatically when contending with larger and more powerful conditions. The last thing I want to do is scare you out of trying. Instead of keeping you stuck on the beach, hopefully you take the initiative to get serious about getting in shape.

In order to smoothly transition to larger waves, try to remember the following suggestions: When you find the wave you want, don't go at it half-heartedly. Commit to catching the wave with every ounce of your being. Anything less, and you will put yourself in a dangerous situation. Take a couple extra strokes when paddling for a bigger wave. Even if you think you are into the wave, this added insurance is often necessary. You might blow the drop, but chances are you will realize that wiping out is not so bad and head back out for more.

Each time you venture into uncharted territory, you expand your threshold. Even if you fail to catch a wave, being in the lineup will make you more comfortable the next time you are faced with similar conditions. The more you push yourself into bigger waves, the easier it becomes to try new maneuvers in smaller surf. Waves will seem to slow down, and you free yourself to take a more playful approach.

Tips for Further Improvement

You might not care about becoming a better surfer. Maybe you are content to catch waves and cruise from Point A to Point B, and that is fine. On the other hand, if progressing is your aim, there are several things you can do to positively impact your surfing ability.

Go surfing . . . Duh! – I realize it is painfully obvious, but the best way to get better at something is to do it a lot. As Malcolm Gladwell explained in his bestselling book *Outliers,* becoming a master of anything requires roughly 10,000 hours of practice.

Get in the movies – I explained the use of video feedback to improve style, but seeing oneself in action works wonders with any aspect of surfing improvement. Why am I falling when I take off? How do I keep losing waves after I catch them? Why can't I get more speed? The answers are all right there on the screen.

Look around you – Watch people surf. Whether you buy a surfing DVD, peruse the Internet for video clips, or pay more attention at your local surf spot, there is plenty to learn from watching other surfers.

Get on board – Never let something so trivial as no beach or no waves impede your surfing progress. Skateboarding, snowboarding, wake-boarding, or mind surfing each provides a worthwhile substitute for the real thing.

Pay your entry fee – Competition is not for everyone, but throwing your hat into the competitive arena forces you to perform. The judges will let you know whether or not your act is working.

Get out of town – Surfing the same spot every day has some benefits, but in order to truly progress it is important to ride different types of waves. Traveling to new spots works on multiple aspects of your surfing. Inevitably, when you return home, you are a better surfer.

Don't be afraid to fall – Remember, it is only water (that is, if you're not surfing over a reef or some rocks). You will fall. I promise. You may as well fall while trying something new rather than doing the same old moves over and over. You will not know what you are capable of until you push yourself.

CHAPTER 13 - ALL THE RIGHT MOVES

In This Chapter
Bottom Turn
Floater
Cutback
Re-Entry
Snap/Slash
Tuberide
Aerial
Riding the Nose

Have you mastered every concept explained in the previous chapter? Have you stood in front of a mirror and practiced your stance? Can you go fast? Do you have a good idea of where to sit in the lineup? Are you ripping, at least in your mind? Okay, we can continue.

In this chapter I will break down the primary maneuvers of surfing from the basic to the radical. By the end, you will understand what it takes to perform each move. You can decide for yourself when you are ready to try them. Better yet, let the wave decide for you. There is a time and place for everything, and it is impossible to impose your will upon a wave. Do not force it, just read the sections and determine the right move for the occasion.

Bottom Turn

If there is one essential move that makes every other maneuver happen, the bottom turn is it. A well-timed arc off the bottom of the wave redirects the board back up the face in preparation for whatever you have in mind. Unfortunately, the bottom turn hardly garners any big glossy photos or scores points in competition and is thus often overlooked. The surfers overlooking it, however, are

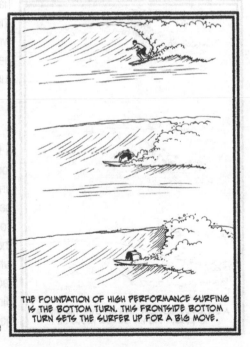

THE FOUNDATION OF HIGH PERFORMANCE SURFING IS THE BOTTOM TURN. THIS FRONTSIDE BOTTOM TURN SETS THE SURFER UP FOR A BIG MOVE.

not accomplishing much on a wave. Without a solid bottom turn, the rest of your ride is mush.

There are several variations on the move, but certain key elements are always present.

Speed up – As with any turn, speed is essential. Without it you will tip over. After a few down-the-line pumps for maximum velocity, pick a spot on the wave where you want to try a move.

Drop to the bottom – Prior to reaching the spot where you want to perform a move, angle down the wave face toward the flats. Be sure to

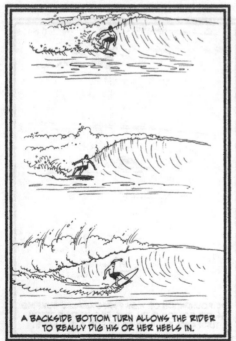

have your feet centered over the stringer. Otherwise you will be off balance and likely never get beyond the bottom turn.

Dip and twist – Once in the flats, dip your shoulder a few inches (rear shoulder for a frontside bottom turn and front shoulder if you are heading backside). Also twist your upper body slightly in the direction you wish to go, which should be back up the face of the wave. Whatever direction your upper body goes, your board will follow.

A BACKSIDE BOTTOM TURN ALLOWS THE RIDER TO REALLY DIG HIS OR HER HEELS IN.

Apply pressure to either your toes or heels, depending on which way you are going (toes for a frontside turn and heels if you are going backside). By dipping, twisting, and employing pressure with the toes or heels, you will redirect back up the wave face.

Spread 'em – Do not put all your weight on your front foot or all on your back foot. Rather, keep your mass distributed equally between the front and back.

Be flexible – Depending upon the situation, you may need to either speed up or slow down your turn. In quick, beachbreak conditions, you will need to snap your bottom turn in order to get back up the face in a hurry. Otherwise the wave will be gone before you can redirect toward the top. In longer, more drawn-out surf, you can extend your bottom turn and project farther down-the-line.

Practice, practice, practice – To really hone your bottom turns, experiment with subtle variations as often as possible. Closeouts do not offer a lot of room for maneuvering, but they provide a great opportunity to practice turning off the bottom.

Do something! – Once you learn to emerge from a bottom turn with speed intact, you are ready for anything. You are a little bird leaving the nest. A vast range of maneuvers awaits, so start trying them. As Young M.C. once said, "Don't just stand there, bust a move!"

Floater

The easiest maneuver to add to one's resumé is the floater, a lateral drifting trip across the lip of a wave. Introduced in the early 1980s, the

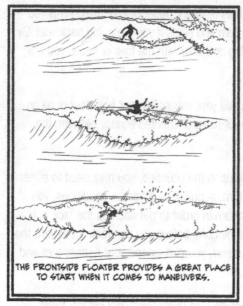

THE FRONTSIDE FLOATER PROVIDES A GREAT PLACE
TO START WHEN IT COMES TO MANEUVERS.

floater is considered both an individual move and a means of traversing across an otherwise un-makeable section in order to reconnect with the open face. While it does not enjoy the sort of high-performance status it warranted during its late '80s heyday, the floater remains a viable component of every surfer's repertoire.

To perform a floater, aim down-the-line and try to pick up some speed. Look for a section that is beginning to crumble ahead of you. Without dropping all the way into the flats, do a partial bottom turn, redirecting just enough to climb the face without going anywhere near vertical. Approach the breaking section at roughly a forty-five-degree angle. At the lip, unweight so you can "float" across the top of the wave. Before expending all of your speed, initiate your descent by twisting your upper body toward the shore. Prepare for landing by slightly bending your knees.

The floater can be tweaked here and there to add some spice, but the real excitement surrounding this move occurs when the stakes are raised. The "dump floater" is a risky move that culminates with a free-fall into the flats. Many a knee and ankle have been injured thanks to botched landings. A floater on a big wave or across a really powerful section still manages to draw hoots from onlookers.

Cutback

The cutback is a gradual, carving, 180-degree change of direction that takes place on the shoulder of a wave and brings the surfer back toward the pocket. I still remember my first cutback. It was an accident. I had been surfing for around a year. I was getting the hang of angling down-the-line and starting to generate some speed. Next thing I know, I am about to turn an innocent

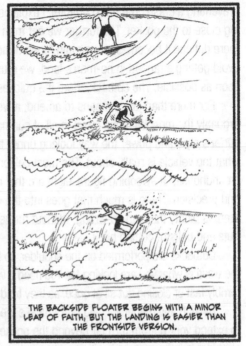

THE BACKSIDE FLOATER BEGINS WITH A MINOR LEAP OF FAITH, BUT THE LANDING IS EASIER THAN THE FRONTSIDE VERSION.

paddler into a bloodied speed bump. Instinct had me instantly shifting my weight to the tail of my board in an effort to slow my forward momentum. At the same time, I involuntarily turned my upper body back from the way in which I had come in hopes of avoiding a collision. In that glorious moment, my surfboard became an extension of my body. (I probably looked like I was throwing my back out, but whatever I did worked.) I avoided the paddler like a slalom skier skirting past a gate, and I inadvertently pulled off a cutback in the process. It was a win-win situation.

Just as the floater enables a surfer to cover a large chunk of down-the-line ground, the cutback also serves a purpose. And it is not just preventing a crash. In the last chapter, I explained the importance of staying close to the pocket. The further we get from this power source, the more difficult it becomes to maintain forward momentum. Therefore, to avoid getting stranded in no-man's land, we must return to the pocket as soon as possible. The cutback offers the quickest road home.

Far more than just a means to an end, a well-executed cutback is arguably the most beautiful move in all of surfing. A cutback lays bare a surfer's style and power the way looking under the hood of a car shows what the vehicle is really about. The most celebrated example is the "roundhouse," a swooping figure-eight arc that requires the utmost control and precision. There is much that goes into the making of a cutback, so there is plenty that can go wrong. Without further ado, let us get into the nuts and bolts of cutting back.

Cutbacks are performed on the shoulder, so the sloping end section of the wave is what you are looking for. You need a wave that is not breaking terribly fast or closing out all at once, as they tend not to have shoulders at all.

As with any maneuver, you gotta have speed. Use your momentum to extend your bottom turn far beyond the pocket. Projection onto the shoulder is important, as it will provide ample turning space. Approach the shoulder, heading up at around a forty-five-degree angle. Let off the gas on the way up and do your best to evenly distribute your weight over your board. Balance will enable you to hold onto your speed throughout the turn. Maintaining speed is best accomplished by bending your knees (to lower your center of gravity) and keeping your arms outstretched. Start your turn by twisting your head and shoulders and dropping your leading shoulder back down the face. By squaring your upper body with the beach, your board will begin its arc. Keep balanced, but apply some pressure to your inside rail. Your leading arm serves as a pivot point, allowing you to guide your board back towards the pocket.

Halfway through the maneuver, it is important to reassess the situation. Is the wave heading off down-the-line without you? If so, you might want to cut it short and try to catch up. To do so, turn your upper body back the other way and shift weight to the opposite rail. If there appears to be enough room to continue the maneuver without losing the wave, keep it going until your board is facing back toward the whitewater. As you approach the whitewater, turn your upper body in the opposite direction and shift your weight to the other rail just before contact. Bank off the whitewater and head into your next move down-the-line.

Try mind-surfing your way through a bunch of cutbacks before making a real-life attempt. Do a few in the street on a skateboard as well. Once you can picture the move and pull it off in your head it should be easier. The most common problem with cutbacks is trying to carve too hard and blowing all your speed. Maintaining weight distribution through the turn is critical. With the right balance, pretty soon you will be banking around the shoulder like a Formula One racer.

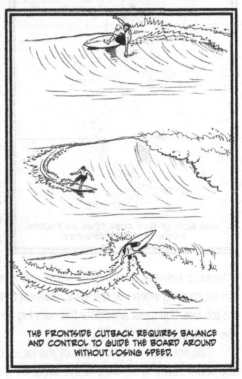

THE FRONTSIDE CUTBACK REQUIRES BALANCE AND CONTROL TO GUIDE THE BOARD AROUND WITHOUT LOSING SPEED.

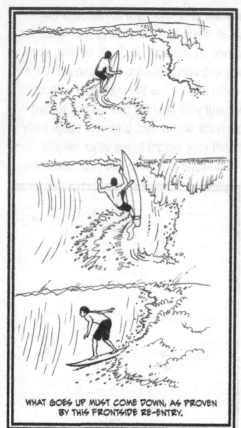

WHAT GOES UP MUST COME DOWN, AS PROVEN
BY THIS FRONTSIDE RE-ENTRY.

Re-Entry

If you are ready to hit the lip, you are leaving the realm of the practical and venturing into the radical. Hopefully, this is not just a symptom of a mid-life crisis; but if so, it is much cheaper than buying a sports car. Alternately referred to as a reo, off-the-lip, off-the-top, lip smack, or lipper, a re-entry can be done on a longboard but thrives on the maneuverability and short turning radius of a short-board or fish.

Since the reo can only be performed in the steep-est section of the wave, there is considerable risk involved. Choosing the opti-mal section makes all the difference between a successful lipper and a belly flop. The lip should not yet be pitching when you decide to attempt a re-entry. If it is, you will likely be too late. You must anticipate the pitching lip and try to get to the top of the wave in time to meet it.

I do not have to remind you of the need for speed, so let us get to the bottom turn. In contrast to the setup for a cutback, you do not want to project onto the shoulder. And unlike with a floater, in this case begin your bottom turn in the flats so you can fully redirect up into the lip. Your bottom turn should angle your board straight up toward the top of the wave. Avoid thinking vertical in the beginning. There will be time for that later. Start slow and work your way up to it. As you begin to ascend, un-weighting will allow you to rise up the wave face. Just before your board hits the cascading lip, apply pressure to the tail and turn your upper body to face back down the wave. Wherever your upper body goes, the board will follow. Your board should bank off the lip and redirect toward the bottom of the wave. Watch the nose on the way down. It is really easy to nosedive after a re-entry. Apply pressure to the tail to keep the nose from burying at the bottom. Look down-the-line and prepare for your next move.

The re-entry has evolved for today's hotshot surfer. A solid reo is still a top-notch maneuver, but to be cutting edge you have to take it a step further. Busting through the lip and sliding the tail of the board around while precariously perched atop the wave has become standard issue for any high-level ripper. This is not much different in theory from a nor-mal re-entry, other than requiring greater balance in order to keep from completely sliding out. Many surfers deliberately extend the slide into a 360-degree turn, known as a "reverse."

Snap/Slash

In the housing market, location is everything. The same goes for surfing maneuvers. There are places on a wave that simply beg for a full roundhouse cutback, and there are places where it will never fit. Closer to the pocket, the cutback is often replaced by its less elegant cousin—the snap. Alternately called a slash, the snap is an abrupt change of direction on a steep section of face that is limited to shortboard surfing. Longboards do not turn rapidly enough, and a fish tends to slide out when jerked around quickly.

Whereas a cutback relies on the rail to carve back towards the pocket, the snap is performed with a heavy dose of tail. Stomping on the back section of the board will cease all forward momentum; therefore, the steepness of the wave is needed to regain speed. The slash happens on a dime.

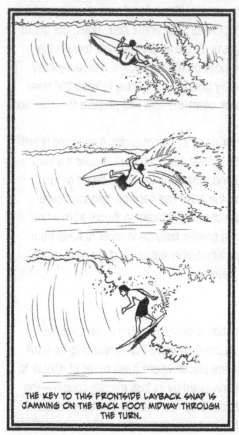

THE KEY TO THIS FRONTSIDE LAYBACK SNAP IS JAMMING ON THE BACK FOOT MIDWAY THROUGH THE TURN.

A normal bottom turn is used to set up the move. Upon reaching the upper half of the wave, begin the snap by simultaneously releasing the weight from your front foot and applying heavy pressure on the back foot. At the same time, turn your upper body back toward the shore. Your board should whip around, and it is up to you to get centered over the board for the descent. Bend your front knee through the snap while straightening the back leg. Try to get your weight forward to regain momentum back down the face and set up another maneuver.

The more committed the snap, the more likely

you are to come to a complete stop. Some snaps can have the reverse effect and actually generate speed. To accomplish a "speed snap," let off the back foot earlier in the turn and reapply pressure to the front foot while still near the top of the wave. This is a good way to set up another turn down-the-line.

A fun variant to the typical slash is the layback snap, sometimes referred to as "dropping the wallet." The legs do the same thing they would for a standard snap, but the upper body twists toward the wave rather than the beach. Since your head turns to look behind you for an instant, it appears as if you have dropped your wallet and are looking for it in your wake. The important part in pulling off a layback snap is to push your board far enough around so that it ends up beneath you. Otherwise, you will fall on your back.

As with the re-entry, modern versions of the snap include a fins-free tail-slide. Again, this adaptation requires amazing balance, control, and wave knowledge to keep from sliding out.

Tuberide

At last, we have come to surfing's ultimate prize, the tube ride. Most aspects of riding waves can be explained in words, but when it comes to riding within the hollow innards of a churning wave, I will not try to tell you what it feels like. I am convinced that nothing in life can compare to this experience. The sensation is indescribable, but I will be happy to break down how it is done.

I suggest first getting acquainted with the tube. You need to understand wave dynamics before attempting to enter the belly of the beast. I am not talking about learning some crazy math formula, just about swimming around and watching waves as they barrel. From there, try bodysurfing inside the tube and eventually try it on a bodyboard. These methods of tuberiding can be performed on much smaller waves and are far easier than doing it while standing atop a surfboard. Practice keeping your eyes open. Blindly going into a tube defeats the purpose. Also, go back to your mirror and practice your tube stance, not to look cool but to make sure you can get into a tight crouched position without any wayward limbs poking out.

In order to get tubed, there must be a tube. It deserves mentioning that a crumbly wave does not pitch, and therefore does not provide a tube. You need a wave that throws as it breaks, creating a hollow void beneath the lip. Also, while a shortboard is the easiest vehicle upon which to get tubed, any board will work.

The set-up is the most difficult part of getting tubed. Once you understand which section of the wave will pitch, the task becomes positioning yourself under the lip while maintaining enough speed to emerge out the other end. Sometimes you must speed up to get in a tube down-the-line, and other times you need to slow down and wait for it. Intentionally slowing your forward momentum is called "stalling" and can be considered a maneuver in itself. If it appears the wave is about to pitch but you will outrun the tube, stalling is like applying the brakes. You stall by sticking your arm in the face of the wave, applying pressure to the tail of the board, or turning into the flats (straightening out) to wait for the wave to jack up. Understand that each of these actions will place you directly in the most dangerous section of the wave, but that is what getting tubed is all about.

Once you have gotten underneath the pitching lip, be sure to stay centered over your board for balance. You will probably need to have your knees bent to fit into the tube, but this also helps to maintain balance and navigate any bumps along the way. Point your front hand out of the tube, and watch where you're going. In the beginning, you will be so excited that you will be unable to think. Eventually, you learn to relax and make adjustments that will help plot a course toward the exit.

Hollow beachbreak waves tend to close-out more often than not, but they provide a perfect opportunity to practice riding the tube. "Pull in," or slot yourself within the barrel, and ride as far as you can. Try to avoid jumping off, because the farther you go, the more energy the wave expends. Therefore, it will not have as

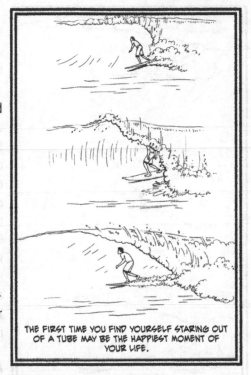

THE FIRST TIME YOU FIND YOURSELF STARING OUT OF A TUBE MAY BE THE HAPPIEST MOMENT OF YOUR LIFE.

much power left at the end to give you a thrashing. And, you might surprise yourself and come shooting out the end unscathed.

At some point you will find yourself innocently plodding along a wave when you hear a paddler bark out, "Pull in!" If you have not already become a tube seeker, here comes your trial by fire. The alternative, straightening out to avoid the falling lip, brands you as a "tube dodger," an unenviable position at the bottom of the totem pole. The choice is yours—pull in or go in.

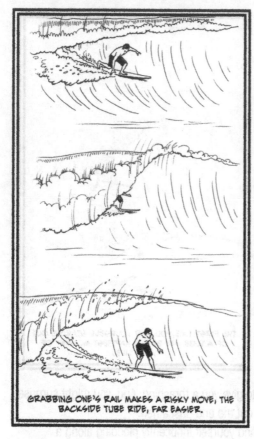

GRABBING ONE'S RAIL MAKES A RISKY MOVE, THE
BACKSIDE TUBE RIDE, FAR EASIER.

As difficult as it is to learn how to ride the tube with proficiency, backside tuberiding proves even more of a challenge. Contorting your body to fit within the confines of the tube while riding backside calls for some awkward positioning. As a result, maintaining speed and balance becomes harder. Grabbing the outside rail with your rear hand and lowering your back knee onto the board, a stance known as "pig-dogging," helps to steady the board.

Aerial

"If man were meant to fly, he would have been born with wings." I don't know who said that, but he is obviously oblivious to the high-flying stunts performed by the latest generation of surfers. Another move that favors the lightness and maneuverability of a shortboard, aerials have revolutionized state-of-the-art surfing. Getting airborne, interestingly enough, is not the biggest challenge. Landing is the hard part.

Since aerials require taking flight, speed is of the essence. Other factors that come in handy are an onshore wind (to help provide lift from the back of the wave) and some "ramps," or small sections of pitching lip that serve as launching pads.

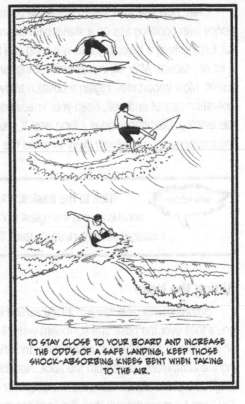

TO STAY CLOSE TO YOUR BOARD AND INCREASE THE ODDS OF A SAFE LANDING, KEEP THOSE SHOCK-ABSORBING KNEES BENT WHEN TAKING TO THE AIR.

Once you gather some speed and locate a ramp down-the-line, do not bother with a full bottom turn. Instead, widen your stance a few inches for extra stability and keep your knees slightly bent. Angle upwards toward the lip and prepare for liftoff. At the lip, un-weight but stay compact to maintain contact with your board. Grabbing one or both rails helps with this keeping attached. Avoid the temptation to go huge in the beginning. A small successful flight is better than a soaring flop, right? Just ask the Wright brothers.

Don't look now, but you are flying! I am not going to leave you hanging. I just wanted you to pause for a second and enjoy the view from up there.

Okay, now use your feet to guide the board back around. Some experience with boosting airs on a skateboard or snowboard is extremely helpful. Establishing a trajectory that will bring you back into the wave will take a lot of practice. After all, waves are moving targets, and each one is different. Most importantly, regain a position above your board. Otherwise this operation cannot end well. Keep your knees bent, and commit to sticking the landing. Confidence goes a long way. If you see yourself riding out of the maneuver, you are more likely to make the subtle adjustments to do so.

"HEY, KOOK!"   **Stick to the basics.** A kook attempting to boost an aerial is among the ugliest sights on earth. Until you have mastered other maneuvers, leave the flying to the experts.

Riding the Nose

Before shortboards revolutionized surfing in the late 1960s, hanging one's toes over the nose of a surfboard was all the rage. The ability to ride on the nose is something of an art form and still draws a firm line separating the competent surfer from the kook. Noseriding remains the ultimate in longboard performance. Ten toes hanging over the nose, a.k.a. "Hanging Ten," are far more difficult than five, and the longer you can stay perched up there, the better.

On a longboard, speed is not an issue. Due to their size, the boards go fast whether you like it or not. Their expanded planing area allows them to get up and go with little effort from the rider. Properly setting up for a noseride is critical. You cannot simply run to the nose at any old time and dangle your tootsies over the end. Try it if you do not believe me. You will nosedive, guaranteed.

The first objective in setting up for a noseride is to get the entire board to the top of the wave and as close to the pocket as possible. This is accomplished by stalling to let the wave roll beneath you. As soon as the wave catches up to you, the next goal is to quickly move to the nose. The distance is around five feet, and you must move gracefully so as not to rock the boat. Try to think like a cat rather than a drunken elephant. Shuffling your feet will get you from Point A to Point B, but it is not pretty.

The ideal way to traverse this space is a stylish dance move of sorts known as "cross-stepping." Remember, your feet are angled at roughly a two-o'clock position (ten-o'clock for goofy-footers). Maintaining this bearing, bring your back foot around and place it directly in front of the other. Next swing what was the front foot back to its natural position in front. One more of these two-steps, and you should arrive at your destination.

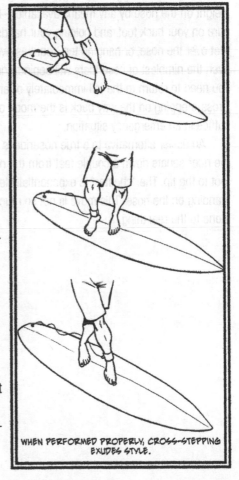

WHEN PERFORMED PROPERLY, CROSS-STEPPING EXUDES STYLE.

Technically, standing anywhere near the front of the board constitutes a noseride, but purists require toes clearly beyond the nose. Getting there is half the battle, and staying for any length of time without burying the nose provides the bigger challenge. Clocking tip time requires keeping your weight off the nose by any means available—leaning back, applying pressure on your back foot, and holding your hands behind you. Dangling both feet over the nose, or hanging ten, requires even more poise. Eventually even the nimblest of noseriders will begin to nosedive. When that happens, you need to return to the tail immediately or endure a certain wipeout. Cross-stepping on the way back is the mode of choice, but shuffling will suffice in an emergency situation.

An easier alternative to a true noseride is the "cheater five," whereby the rider squats down a couple feet from the nose and extends his front foot to the tip. The "cheater" is exponentially less demanding than actually standing on the nose. This move is not so much kooky as it is a stepping-stone to the real thing.

PART V: ORGANIZED SURFING

CHAPTER 14 - ENTER TO WIN

In This Chapter

Ups and Downs of Competition

Soul Man or Sellout

Rules

Scoring

Tips for Success

Surfing differs from mainstream sports in many respects, not the least of which is the notion of competition. With any "ball" sport, or most other athletic endeavors, someone is always keeping score or keeping track of time. The overwhelming majority of surfing occurs without parameters of any kind. Only a fraction of the surfing population ever takes part in competition. Nevertheless, contests regularly occur at surfing beaches around the world. The best surfers earn a large portion of their living from competing, and thousands of weekend warriors engage in local competitions every chance they get.

Surf contests are not for everyone, but they are alive and well. Chances are, there is a contest in your neighborhood with a division made just for you. In this chapter, we deconstruct surf competition to find out if there is a trophy topped with a little metal surfer in your future.

Ups and Downs of Competition

As great as it is to surf for pure enjoyment, no surfer would voluntarily decline the opportunity to surf for a living if given the chance. Let's see, travel the world and get paid to ride great waves, or strap on a tie and sit in a stuffy cubicle in front of a computer screen every day. Hmm, what to do, what to do? We can agree that there is no better job on the planet than professional surfer. For an aspiring pro, local amateur contests provide the primary means for getting noticed. There are pro surfers that do not compete, but you can count them on your fingers, and even these guys came up through the amateur ranks as youngsters.

For successful competitive surfers, the ultimate goal is to compete at the pro level. However, competition provides many benefits aside from a path to the pros. Contests can make you a better surfer. Obviously, the goal is to win. If you pay attention to the reasons you fail to advance in a contest and focus on correcting these mistakes, you will improve as a surfer. Maybe you are choosing crappy waves, or you are falling every time you stand up, or your style resembles that of a primate. Whatever it is, you will need to fix it if you want to succeed in competition.

Another great thing about events such as these is the people you meet. Some of my best friends today are folks I first met at surf contests twenty-five years ago. A gathering of the tribes puts you in contact with lots of people who share common interests. You might not love everyone, but if you are looking for some new surf buddies, this is as good a place as any to start.

And since surf competition clearly falls under the heading of sport, another benefit is learning about sportsmanship. How to win with humility, lose with dignity, and have fun either way are important life lessons. Especially for kids who are not into team sports, surf contests offer exposure to these concepts. And if improving your surfing, making friends, and learning about sportsmanship are not enough to spark your interest, consider the prospect of bragging rights and some pretty cool prizes.

"HEY, KOOK!"   **This is supposed to be fun, remember?**
Surf contests sometimes earn a reputation for bringing out the worst in people. Overly aggressive stage parents, judging discrepancies, and petty disputes fueled by poor sportsmanship seem to find their way into competition of any sort. Surf events are not immune to these evils. As long as you opt for the high road and keep the focus on fun, these types of incidents cannot spoil your experience.

Soul Man or Sellout

The notion of "soul surfing" arose as the antithesis to professionalism in the mid-1970s. Competition and the budding surf industry faced a backlash for exploiting surfing's purity for monetary gain. Seeking fame and fortune from riding waves, the purists insisted, perverted the sport. These soul surfers rode for the intrinsic value of communing with nature. The dichotomy has remained a part of surfing. Supposedly, you are on one side of the fence or the other.

Perception, it turns out, often trumps reality. For instance, Tom Curren was hailed by soul and non-soul surfers alike while competing to three world championships and earning a great deal of money from sponsors. For some reason, he was never viewed as a sellout, despite making a healthy living from the sport.

Seeing as how the great majority of surfers take part in the pursuit of riding waves for nothing other than personal enjoyment, the entire concept of "soul surfing" seems a little silly. We are basically all in this for the same reasons. Some are just lucky and dedicated enough to make a living from it. Soul surfer, competitor, or just plain surfer, it does not really matter.

Rules

A surfing competition can be a confusing circus of activity for the uninitiated. There are horns blaring, flags waving, and people running in and out of the water every few minutes. To try and make the whole spectacle a bit less bewildering, here are some basic rules to help make sense of it all.

Divisions – Contests are typically broken down into divisions based on age (11 and under, 12–14, 15–17, 18–24, 25–34, and so on), type of board (shortboard, longboard, bodyboard, etc.), and sometimes skill level (novice, advanced, pro).

Heats – Each division, depending on the number of contestants, is separated into heats, much like with a swim meet. Heats may be fifteen or twenty minutes, and there are four or six surfers per heat. Each surfer is given a colored singlet, or Lycra rashguard, to wear while surfing so the judges can differentiate between the competitors.

Timing – The heat begins with a horn blow and the raising of a green flag. Surfers may paddle out at this time unless it has been established that they may do so earlier based on surf conditions. With five minutes remaining, there is another horn blow and a yellow flag is raised. At the end of the heat, the horn blows yet again, and the green flag signifies the start of the next heat (or a red flag indicates a stoppage

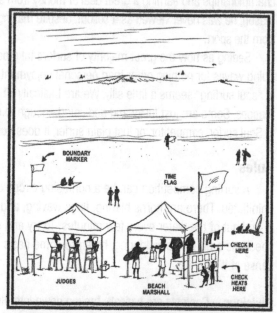

SURF CONTESTS RANGE FROM NOTHING MORE THAN A CARD TABLE AND HORN TO SOMETHING CLOSE TO A THREE-RING CIRCUS AND EVERYTHING IN BETWEEN.

of competition). If you ride a wave after your heat has ended, you may be penalized.

Boundaries — Contest organizers will use flags on the beach to delineate the area competitors are allowed to surf during their heat. Ideally, all recreational surfers stay out of the competition area.

Wave Count — During a heat, there is a maximum number of waves each surfer is allowed to ride, usually ten. Any more than that and a penalty may be assessed. Each ride becomes official when the surfer's hands leave the rails upon standing up. A surfer's best two rides are tallied to determine his final placing.

Advancement — In most contests, there is 50 percent advancement from each round. When there are only four or six surfers remaining, those surfers compete in a final heat, which is usually a little longer than the earlier heats.

Interference — One competitor is not allowed to interfere with another surfer's scoring potential. An interference penalty is assessed when one surfer drops in on another. Snaking is a no-no. Also, you cannot intentionally paddle in front of another surfer or you will be penalized. Interference rules vary depending on the nature of the waves, such as predominant rights, lefts, or random peaks scattered along the beach.

Scoring

A judging panel consists of three to five (hopefully) competent and unbiased arbiters of surfing prowess. Scoring is subjective, so the judges may have varying opinions on the same ride. Sometimes these judges are trained professionals, but at small grassroots events you may get a few stragglers who just happened to be hanging around the beach. These guys determine whether or not you make it through a heat. If you accidentally snaked one of them the other day, chances are you are out of luck. They wield the ultimate power.

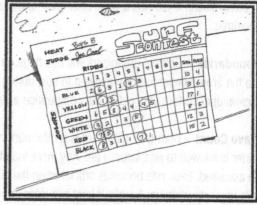

WHEN COMPETING, BE SURE TO CHECK THE JUDGING SHEETS FOR TABULATION ERRORS.

The job of a judge can be difficult. Sometimes all six surfers are up and riding at once, or perhaps the conditions are dreadful and no surfer is able to separate himself from the pack. The judge watches every ride and assigns each a value. The criteria read something like this: "A surfer must perform radical controlled maneuvers in the critical section of the wave with speed, power, and flow to maximize scoring potential. Innovative/progressive surfing as well as variety of repertoire will be taken into consideration when awarding points for waves ridden."

Each judge awards a score between one and ten points (ten being a perfect score) for each wave ridden. Some use half-point increments, and some break it down even further into tenths of a point. In some larger events, computers are used that allow scores to be quickly averaged and announced soon after they happen. Without computer scoring, judging sheets are manually tabulated after each heat, so it takes ten minutes or more to find out how everyone fared. Either way, the results are soon announced and/or posted on a heat board.

Tips for Success

A perennial knock on competition is that the best surfer does not always win. Talent helps, but it takes much more than mere surfing ability to come out on top. Surf contests are often wave-catching contests as much as anything else. Without getting waves during your heat, it does not matter if you are the greatest surfer to ever step foot on a surfboard. You are not going to win. With that in mind, here are a few tips for becoming a better competitor:

Watch and learn – Sit on the beach and watch several heats. Notice different approaches taken by competitors and decide on a strategy you plan to implement.

Stay active – Do not sit there and wait for a gift from above. The best competitors are like sharks, always prowling the lineup in search of waves.

Assume the position – By studying the conditions prior to surfing, you can determine the best place to be in order to catch a set wave. The other competitors will want to catch the best waves as well, so it is up to you to get the inside track.

Don't repeat your mistakes – You can't win 'em all. When you lose, there is a reason. Your wave selection was poor, you surfed too conservatively, you paddled out at the wrong beach—the cause for your bad showing could be anything. Whatever it is, pinpoint where things went wrong and determine not to repeat that mistake again. Eventually, you can eliminate the errors and finish on top.

Worry about yourself – I often overhear young competitors lamenting that they have to surf against So-and-So. Remember, So-and-So might be the best surfer around, but he still has to paddle out and catch waves to win. Good competitors beat good surfers all the time.

Look alive – Regardless of the conditions, judges do not like pessimists. Maintain a positive attitude and make the most of the waves you catch. Flipping the bird to an uncooperative wave will definitely not get you through any heats.

CHAPTER 15 - THROUGH THE RANKS

In This Chapter
Amateur Competition
Professional Surfing
Sponsorship
A Spectator's Guide

You have learned to surf, mastered all sorts of maneuvers, and competed in some contests. Your next step is to breeze through amateur competition, turn pro, and take on the world. I feel like a proud parent sending his child off to college. Before you go, I will offer a few (hundred) words on what you might encounter along the way. Don't forget to thank me when you accept your first world title.

Amateur Competition

If you are serious about competitive surfing, the next step is to get involved in one of the many amateur organizations that conduct contests. Amateur surfers pay an annual membership fee to whichever of the associations they join as well as entry fees for each event. These associations are typically divided into districts. Each district holds local events whereby competitors accrue points throughout the year based on their results. Winners receive trophies and occasionally some surf-related prizes, but the ultimate goal is a high year-end ranking. At season's end, the top competitors from each division are invited to compete in a regional championship, followed by (depending on the size of the organization) a coast-wide or national championship.

Amateur surfers of yesteryear were strictly forbidden from receiving money from either endorsements or contest winnings. Some kids tested the bylaws and were forced to surrender their amateur status. The only way around these rules was to apply money to a fund used exclusively for surf-related travel. These days the line between amateur and professional is blurred. Amateur surfers enjoy the best of both worlds. They still compete in amateur competition, yet their endorsement deals and prize-winnings are rarely questioned.

Professional Surfing

The notion of earning a living by riding a surfboard remained a pipe dream well into the 1970s. There were a number of pro events prior to the formation of a world tour in '76, but it took a governing body and a series of related events to make the fantasy a reality. Since that time, professional surfing has expanded exponentially. More than a thousand humans can legitimately call themselves pro surfers, meaning they either get paid from sponsors or compete for prize money or a combination of the two.

Anyone can be a pro surfer. All you need to do is go online, fill out an entry form for a professional event, plunk down your credit card, and show up at the beach in time for your heat. Congratulations, you are a pro. You are not getting paid, but your friends and the girl you meet at the bar do not need to know that.

Professional surfing can be viewed as a pyramid. At the bottom you have the small local pro events, which have no affiliation with the Association of Surfing Professionals (ASP), the governing body of the sport. Next up is the ASP's World Qualifying Series, a string of events around the globe that are rated based on their prize purse. The smallest events are one-stars, and the largest qualifying contests are six-stars. Points are awarded at each event, with the biggest cash purses doling out the most points. At the culmination of each season, the surfers who have earned the most points on the Qualifying Series rise up the pyramid to the ASP World Tour. This elite level consists of the top thirty-four men and top fifteen women on earth. Each year, they compete in a series of events held at many of the world's most coveted surfing destinations. The top two-thirds of the World Tour surfers at season's end retain their spots for the following season, while the other one-third get replaced by Qualifying Series standouts. The surfer with the most World Tour points at year's end sits atop the entire pyramid as world champion.

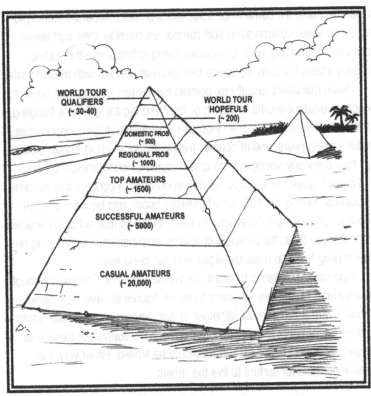

WORLD TOUR
QUALIFIERS
(~ 30-40)

WORLD TOUR
HOPEFULS
(~ 200)

DOMESTIC PROS
(~ 500)

REGIONAL PROS
(~ 1000)

TOP AMATEURS
(~ 1500)

SUCCESSFUL AMATEURS
(~ 5000)

CASUAL AMATEURS
(~ 20,000)

THE VAST MAJORITY OF COMPETITIVE SURFERS NEVER RISE ABOVE THE BOTTOM
FLOOR OF THIS PYRAMID.

Sponsorship

A sponsor provides an athlete with anything from a sticker, to some free clothes, to a monthly check in exchange for the endorsement of their products. Companies within as well as outside the surfing industry dedicate a large part of their marketing efforts to creating teams of sponsored surfers. The rationale for sponsoring athletes is ultimately money. High-profile continents a year for weeks at a stretch proves time consuming and cost is prohibitive. Fortunately, there are other ways to keep track of the tour.

Each World Tour event, as well as many Qualifying Series contests, is webcast live in streaming video and can be found at the organization's website, www.aspworldtour.com. The entire ordeal, from the first heat to the last, can be viewed in the comfort of your home as long as you have a decent computer with a high-speed internet connection. Other than the occasional technical glitch, the simulcasts run smoothly even from the most remote of locations in the middle of the ocean. These webcasts have drawn hundreds of thousands of watchers at one time. Therefore, sponsors use this opportunity to launch a barrage of banner ads and short commercials during lulls in the action.

If you are fortunate enough to watch a World Tour event in person, the experience is often a memorable one, but to the unpredictability of Mother Nature, conditions are not always sono, and eight to ten hours of watching anything becomes burdensome, however, the surfers' remarkable talent creates a spectacle even in marginal surf. The difference between a top level pro and the rest of the surfing world is a chasm. Just as most cyclists would not be able to finish the Tour De France course even if they had a year to do it, most surfers would be overwhelmed by the waves these athletes thrive in. In good conditions, the top pros throw themselves into death defying situations that boggle the mind.

Depending on the event, pro contests allow varying degrees of access to the competitors. Some crowded beaches require security forces, competitors-only areas, and little opportunity for so much as an autograph. On the other hand, events held in remote locations present few barriers between spectators and competitors. In these out-of-the-way settings, spectators can find themselves face-to-face with the best in the world while surfing, dining, or cruising around the contest site.

PART VI: APPENDICES
APPENDICES

APPENDICES

Appendix C: Global Shit-O-Dex

APPENDIX A: HANGIN' NINE

9 Essential Surf Trips

Oahu – This tropical island has something for everyone, from the playful rollers at surfing's birthplace of Waikiki, to the North Shore big wave Mecca, and everything in between.

Southern California – Everyone here surfs, whether it's the Surf City mayhem of Huntington Beach, the longboard styling of Malibu, or the high-performance capital of Trestles.

Gold Coast Oz – A journey Down Under isn't complete without the epic right-hand point perfection of The Superbank.

East Coast Hurricane Chaser – There's no comparing the thrill of this hunt and the possibility of scoring great waves along a coast that isn't known for surf.

Jeffreys Bay – This quaint surf town was built around the classic right-hand point of the same name.

Indonesia boat trip – Drop anchor at your own private reef complete with a personal chef, air-conditioned bunk, and an unforgettable adventure with your best mates.

Caribbean – Time slows to a crawl the moment you step off the plane, and the playful warm water reefs offer the ultimate antidote to winter.

Central America – From the jungles settings of Costa Rica to the Mexican Pipeline at Puerto Escondido, Latin America provides mucho waves and a number of inexpensive alternatives.

Europe – It's hard to beat the Old World charm of surfing hollow beachbreaks alongside five-hundred-year-old castles, and you can even surf in the nude.

9 Surfers You Should Know (Other than Duke and Gidget)

Greg "Da Bull" Noll – This outspoken pioneer of big-wave surfing led the '50s attack of California transplants on Oahu's deadliest waves.

Miki Dora – The Malibu iconoclast was legendary for his attitude as much as his stylish longboard surfing.

Gerry Lopez – Synonymous with the world's most revered wave, Mr. Pipeline casually set the standard for tuberiding in the '70s.

Larry "Rubberman" Bertlemann – This innovative Hawaiian launched New School surfing soon after the advent of the short surfboard.

Mark Richards – The great MR was the first pro surfing dynasty, claiming four consecutive world titles for Australia from 1979–1982.

Tom Curren – This savior of California surfing was widely recognized as a style god as he effortlessly earned three world titles.

Lisa Andersen – The four-time world champ from Florida reinvented women's surfing with a combination of beauty, grace, and power.

Kelly Slater – From humble roots in Florida to an unprecedented eleven world titles, he is the Michael Jordan, Tiger Woods, and Lance Armstrong of surfing.

Laird Hamilton – Constantly searching for the 100-foot wave, this tow surfing pioneer might be leading surfers off the edge of the earth.

9 Stupid Surfing Questions (That Aren't Stupid)

- Do those suits really keep you warm?
- What's in the bag, a dead body?
- Why don't they put an engine on the back?
- What's the biggest wave you've ever ridden?
- What if you have to use the bathroom?
- Can you surf in the rain?
- Can you surf in the eye of a hurricane?
- May I borrow your favorite surfboard?
- Which side does the wax go on?

9 Challenges Facing the Sport

- Deadbeat image
- Death of the craftsmen
- Reef destruction
- Crowding
- Beach access
- Pollution
- Surf shop extinction
- Matthew McConaughey
- Kooks

9 Signs That You Might Be a Kook...

- You think a flyaway kickout is a legitimate maneuver
- You drive around with a board on the roof but don't surf
- You wear your leash all the way back to your car after a session
- Your email address includes some variant on the word "surf"
- You wear a rashguard or wetsuit anywhere other than to the beach
- You have a "Team" sticker on your board
- You always ask your buddy if he saw your last wave
- You quit surfing because "It's too damn crowded" or "It just doesn't get good anymore"
- You worry about whether or not you're a kook rather than just going surfing

Appendix B: Surfspeak

aerial: maneuver in which a surfer launches off the lip and into the air

agro: exercising an aggressive approach to catching and/or riding waves
The after-work crowd is pretty aggro

airbrush: tool used for applying paint to a shaped surfboard blank prior to glassing; the process of applying such paint

backdoor: to take off from a position behind the peak of a wave

backside/backhand: riding with one's back to the wave as opposed to facing it

backwash: a wave returning to the ocean after washing up a steep beach

bail/bail out: to voluntarily abandon one's surfboard during a ride

beachbreak: waves that break over a sandbar

blank: the foam core of a surfboard

boardshorts: bathing suit designed for surfing, also called trunks, baggies, boardies

boil: an area of turbulence in the face of a wave caused by rock or coral near the surface

booties: neoprene rubber shoes designed for surfing in cold water

bottom turn: a redirection at the base of a wave that sends a surfer back up the face

bowl: a steep, powerful, crescent-shaped or concave section of wave face; when a wave forms such a section, that wave bowled up on the inside

breaking: when a wave slows over shallow water and the top collapses forward to create whitewater; what a wave must do in order to be ridden

carve: to turn a surfboard gradually by applying pressure with the toes or heels; to turn powerfully

caught inside: the unenviable position of being shoreward of breaking waves and unable to make it outside

channel: deep-water area void of breaking waves; entry/exit location adjacent to lineup

cheater five: hanging five the easy way; crouching a couple feet from the nose and stretching one's front foot to the tip

choppy: jumbled, difficult to ride surf conditions caused by stiff onshore winds; blown-out

clean: smooth, glassy surf conditions groomed by offshore winds

closeout: a wave that breaks all at once, not good for surfing

continental shelf: shallow, gradually sloping area of the seafloor that begins at the shore and extends seaward; an extended shelf such as that found along the US. East Coast slows and diminishes swell before it reaches the shore

cross-stepping: stylish, foot-over-foot walk toward the nose of a longboard

cutback: 180-degree change of direction executed by a surfer

dawn patrol: early morning surf session

delamination: on a surfboard, the separation of fiberglass from its foam core due to water seepage, a damaging condition that is costly to repair

dig a rail: a surfing blunder whereby the side of the board becomes inadvertently buried beneath the surface, often resulting in a wipeout

ding: any crack, dent, or hole in the fiberglass shell of a surfboard

down-the-line: portion of unbroken wave face beyond where a surfer is riding

double-up: a steeper and more powerful wave formed with the merger of two smaller waves

drag: a surfboard's resistance to forward motion

drive: a surfboard's propensity for generating down-the-line momentum

drop: a surfer's initial downward movement upon catching a wave

drop in: to take off in front of another surfer, an especially offensive maneuver; also to snake

duck dive: technique of submerging beneath an approaching wave while paddling in order to avoid a direct impact

epoxy: stronger and lighter resin than standard fiberglass, more expensive and difficult to work with

face: unbroken surface on the front of a wave; the part of a wave used for surfing

fade: when surfing, to angle in the opposite direction a wave is breaking in order to relocate to a position closer to the pocket

fiberglass: glass fibers woven into cloth that forms the protective outer shell of a surfboard

fin: rudder-like protrusion (or protrusions) on the bottom of a surfboard that provides stability and drive

fin box: base into which fins are attached to a surfboard

fish: a short, wide, board, usually with two fins and a rounded nose, that originated in the 1970s and has since reemerged as a great small-wave board design

flat: ocean condition void of wave activity

flats: area ahead of a breaking wave

floater: surfing maneuver where the rider traverses laterally across the top of a breaking section of wave

foam: polyurethane core of a surfboard; see also whitewater

foil: a surfboard's flow of thickness as viewed from a cross-section

freak set: an unexpected group of large waves, also called a sneaker set or cleanup set

freeboarding: the act of surfing on a boat's wake while being pulled along holding a tow rope

freefall: to drop through the air from the top to the bottom of a wave

frontside or forehand: riding while facing toward a wave as opposed to with one's back to the wave

fullsuit: a wetsuit that extends to the wrists and ankles

funboard: an easy-to-ride hybrid surfboard approximately seven to eight inches in length with a rounded nose, usually ridden by older surfers or beginners

glass off: with surf conditions, to become cleaner as a result of lessening winds

glass-on: a fin that is permanently affixed to a board with fiberglass

goofyfoot: a surfer who rides with right foot forward

grommet: a young surfer, also called a gremmie, rat, or menehune

groundswell: waves generated by an offshore weather system as opposed to local winds

gun: a long, tapered surfboard used for riding big waves

hang five: to ride with one foot (five toes) perched over the nose of the board

hang ten: to ride with both feet (ten toes) perched over the nose of the board

haole: any non-Hawaiian, usually a pale-skinned visitor

head-high: waves that measure as tall as their rider, the standard for surf to be considered good

hot dog: outdated term for progressive surfing

Huey: the god of surf who is said to deliver waves

ice cream headache: a brain-freeze brought on by being immersed in extremely cold water

impact zone: area of breaking waves, not a safe place to be

inside: area between breaking waves and the shore

jetty: a rock, steel, or cement structure protruding into the ocean

Kahuna: imaginary Hawaiian surfing god

kick out: to intentionally end a ride by turning and exiting a wave in a seaward direction

knee paddle: to stroke through the water in a kneeling position atop a longboard

kook: an inexperienced or disrespectful surfer

laminate: to apply resin to a shaped surfboard blank

late takeoff: the act of catching a wave that is already breaking

leash: polyurethane safety strap that keeps a surfer attached to his surfboard

left: as viewed from the lineup facing the shore, a wave with unbroken face to the left

lineup: the takeoff area of a surf spot

lip: a section of wave face that is in the process of pitching or plunging

longboard: a surfboard measuring around nine feet or more in length that is generally ridden in the stylish, flowing manner perfected during the 1960s

longshore current: water flowing parallel to shore

lull: an extended period of lessened wave activity between sets

morning sickness: an ugly, uninviting state of the surf prior to grooming by offshore winds

mushy: a weak, sloped wave; also burger or mush burger

nose: the front section of a surfboard

noseride: to stand on the front section of a surfboard while riding a wave

offshore wind: air flow emanating from the shore and blowing toward the sea, creates clean conditions

onshore wind: air flow emanating from the sea and blowing toward the shore, creates choppy conditions

outline: the perimeter shape of a surfboard

outside: anywhere beyond the breaking waves; also called out the back

over the falls: the undesirable predicament of wiping out and being embedded in the cascading lip, resulting in a violent underwater beating

overgunned: riding a surfboard that is disproportionately long for the surf conditions, therefore difficult to turn

party wave: when everyone in the lineup takes off on a single wave

peak: the highest point of an unbroken wave, usually the ideal takeoff position

peaky: surf conditions where waves are exceptionally short, consisting only of peaks and shoulders, the opposite of "walled"

pearl: to bury the nose, usually on takeoff, resulting in a wipeout; also called nosedive

pecking order: established wave-catching order in the lineup, based on seniority or surfing ability

planing surface: area on the bottom of a surfboard that is in almost constant contact with, or planes across, the water

pocket: area of wave face that is closest to the breaking portion of the wave, the steepest and most critical part of the wave

pointbreak: a wave that bends along a headland or point or into a bay, allowing for a long ride

popout: an inexpensive surfboard mass-produced from a mold on a production line as opposed to being hand-shaped

post-session nasal drip: an unexpected release of seawater from the sinuses occurring minutes to a few hours after a surf session

prone out: while surfing, to go from a standing position to lying on one's belly and ride directly to shore

pull in: to get inside the tube; also an encouraging directive yelled by someone paddling to a surfer who is riding ("Pull in!")

pump: to work the surfboard back and forth in an effort to generate down-the-line speed

quiver: a collection of surfboards, usually of varying designs in order to accommodate a range of surf conditions

radical: of a high degree of difficulty; extreme; also rad

rail: the rounded perimeter of a surfboard

rashguard: a snug-fitting Lycra jersey worn to prevent stomach/chest rash from lying atop a surfboard or armpit/neck rash from wearing a wetsuit, also provides protection from sun exposure

re-entry: a radical change of direction performed at the lip of a wave; also reo, off-the-lip, off-the-top

reefbreak: a surf spot that breaks over a coral or rock reef

reform: a breaking wave that had broken previously before dying out in deeper water (I caught a nice little reform on the inside.); the act of a wave breaking again after dying out (That wave reformed on the inside.)

resin: a syrupy coat of fiberglass that is poured over fiberglass cloth and hardens to create a board's outer shell

rideable: the state of being surfable; a wave's capacity for being ridden

right: as viewed from the lineup facing the shore, a wave with unbroken face to the right and whitewater to the left

rip: to demonstrate great skill in riding waves (Did you see that girl out there? She was ripping!); also shred or shralp

rip current: a stream of water flowing out to sea

rocker: the gradual curve of a surfboard as viewed in profile

roller coaster: to ride up and down the wave face while surfing down-the-line

roundhouse: a figure-eight cutback

sandbar: an underwater mound of sand that causes waves to break

section: part of a wave that is in the process of breaking

set: a series of waves that are larger than the average for a given day, typically arriving in groups of two to five but potentially more

shaka: a hand signal whereby the thumb and pinky are extended and other fingers closed, signifying a friendly acknowledgement common among Hawaiian surfers

shoot the pier: to ride a wave between the pilings of a pier

shorebreak: waves that abruptly break in shallow water close to shore, also called shorepound

shortboard: a lightweight, high-performance surfboard averaging around six feet in length

shoulder: sloping, unbroken portion of a wave located beyond the pocket

sideshore wind: wind that blows parallel to the waves; sometimes called devil wind as it can quickly ruin surf conditions

slab: an extremely abrupt, powerful wave breaking atop a shallow reef

snap: a sudden change of direction performed on the face of a wave by applying pressure to the tail

soul surfer: a non-competitive surfer

spin out/slide out: to lose control of one's surfboard due to the fins and tail lifting out of the water

spit: forceful spray emanating from a tube, often propelling a surfer out of the tube and onto the safety of the shoulder

stall: to intentionally slow one's momentum in order to obtain a better position on a wave

stoked: really happy; thrilled

stringer: wooden strip along the center of a surfboard providing strength

surf knots/surf bumps: lumps appearing on a surfer's knees, shins, or tops of feet as a result of knee-paddling

surf sacrifice: ceremonial burning of a surfboard to appease wave gods, usually performed on the beach

surf-up: the movement of popping up on a surfboard from a prone position to standing

surf's up: outdated declaration of quality surf conditions

surfer's ear: excess bony growth in the ear canal brought on by exposure to cold water; also called exostosis

swell: unbroken wave energy travelling across a body of water

switch-foot: to surf in the opposite of one's normal stance, i.e., a regular-foot riding goofy

tail: the rear end of a surfboard

takeoff: the beginning of a ride

tandem: two surfers riding together on one surfboard

three-sixty: a maneuver in which a surfer rotates the board 360 degrees either by carving or sliding

thruster: three-finned shortboard design developed in 1981 by Australian pro surfer Simon Anderson and still in common use today

tides: periodic rise and fall of sea level caused by the earth's rotation and the gravitational pull of the moon

tow-in surfing: mode of catching waves by being pulled along by a personal watercraft and holding a tow rope

trim: state of optimal positioning on the face a wave

tube: the hollow, cylindrical space within a breaking wave; surfing's most coveted destination; also called barrel

turtle turn: when paddling, to roll over with one's board in order to avoid the impact of an oncoming wave

undergunned: riding a surfboard that is disproportionately short for the surf conditions, therefore difficult to keep from sliding out

upwelling: cold water rising to the ocean's surface due to offshore winds that push warmer upper layer out to sea

victory-at-sea: extremely stormy surf conditions caused by strong onshore winds

wahine: a female surfer; also betty

walled: unfavorable, closed out surf conditions

waterman: a person who is comfortable in any surf conditions

wave hog: surfer who catches more than an equitable share of the waves

wave knowledge: an understanding of wave dynamics as it relates to surfing

wax: sticky substance rubbed on the deck of a surfboard to aid in traction

whitecaps: small windblown waves in open waters that topple and disappear

whitewater: broken part of a wave characterized by turbulence and white, foamy water; also soup

windswell: waves generated by local winds as opposed to offshore storm systems

wipe out: to fall off one's surfboard

APPENDIX C: GLOBAL SURF-O-DEX

Magazines

Surfer (USA) – www.surfermag.com

Surfing (USA) – www.surfingmagazine.com

Transworld Surf (USA) – www.surf.transworld.net

The Surfers Journal (USA) – www.surfersjournal.com

Tracks (Australia) – www.tracksmag.com

Australian Surfing Life (Australia) – www.surfinglife.com.au

Stab (Australia) – www.stabmag.com

Transworld Surf Business – www.surf.transworld.net

The Surfer's Path (UK) – www.surferspath.mpora.com

Surf Europe (Europe) – www.surfeurop.mpora.com

Drift (Europe) – www.driftmagazine.co.uk

Zigzag (South Africa) – www.zigzag.co.za

Mundo Rad (USA/Puerto Rico) – www.mundorad.com

Free Surf Hawaii (USA/Hawaii) – www.freesurfmagazine.com

Eastern Surf (USA/East Coast) – www.easternsurf.com

Websites

Surfline.com – Surf cams, reports, forecasts, news

Magicseaweed.com – Surf reports and forecasts

Surfermag.com/surf-reports-and-forecasts/ – Surf reports and forecasts

Stormsurf.com – Surf reports and forecasts

Surfingmagazine.com/swellwatch/ – Surf reports

Aspworldtour.com – Professional competition

Surfersvillage.com – Surf news

Boardfolio.com – Directory

Shop-eat-surf.com – Surf industry news

Organizations
Surf Industry Manufacturer's Association – 949-366-1164, www.sima.com
Surfrider Foundation – 949-492-8170, www.surfrider.org
Surf Aid International – 760-931-1199, www.surfaidinternational.org
Save the Waves Coalition – 831-426-6169, www.savethewaves.org
Reef Check – 310-230-2371, www.reefcheck.org
Surfing Australia – www.surfingaustralia.com
Surfers Against Sewage – www.sas.org.uk
National Scholastic Surfing Association – 714-378-0899, www.nssa.org
Surfing America – 949-276-4660, www.surfingamerica.org
Eastern Surfing Association – 757-233-1790, www.surfesa.org
Western Surfing Association – 949-369-6677, www.surfwsa.org
Hawaiian Surfing Association – 808-638-4267, www.hasasurf.org
International Surfing Association – 858-551-8580, www.isasurf.org
Black Surfing Association – 805-237-1150, www.blacksurfingassociation.com
Surfer's Medical Association – 831-684-0916, www.surfersmedicalassociation.org
Groundswell Society – www.groundswellsociety.org